T0226896

Sleep Apnea

Editors

MARIA V. SUURNA
OFER JACOBOWITZ

OTOLARYNGOLOGIC CLINICS OF NORTH AMERICA

www.oto.theclinics.com

Consulting Editor
SUJANA S. CHANDRASEKHAR

June 2020 • Volume 53 • Number 3

ELSEVIER

1600 John F. Kennedy Boulevard • Suite 1800 • Philadelphia, Pennsylvania, 19103-2899

http://www.oto.theclinics.com

OTOLARYNGOLOGIC CLINICS OF NORTH AMERICA Volume 53, Number 3
June 2020 ISSN 0030-6665, ISBN-13: 978-0-323-73290-1

Editor: Stacy Eastman
Developmental Editor: Laura Fisher

© **2020 Elsevier Inc. All rights reserved.**

This periodical and the individual contributions contained in it are protected under copyright by Elsevier, and the following terms and conditions apply to their use:

Photocopying
Single photocopies of single articles may be made for personal use as allowed by national copyright laws. Permission of the Publisher and payment of a fee is required for all other photocopying, including multiple or systematic copying, copying for advertising or promotional purposes, resale, and all forms of document delivery. Special rates are available for educational institutions that wish to make photocopies for non-profit educational classroom use. For information on how to seek permission visit www.elsevier.com/permissions or call: (+44) 1865 843830 (UK)/(+1) 215 239 3804 (USA).

Derivative Works
Subscribers may reproduce tables of contents or prepare lists of articles including abstracts for internal circulation within their institutions. Permission of the Publisher is required for resale or distribution outside the institution. Permission of the Publisher is required for all other derivative works, including compilations and translations (please consult www.elsevier.com/permissions).

Electronic Storage or Usage
Permission of the Publisher is required to store or use electronically any material contained in this periodical, including any article or part of an article (please consult www.elsevier.com/permissions). Except as outlined above, no part of this publication may be reproduced, stored in a retrieval system or transmitted in any form or by any means, electronic, mechanical, photocopying, recording or otherwise, without prior written permission of the Publisher.

Notice
No responsibility is assumed by the Publisher for any injury and/or damage to persons or property as a matter of products liability, negligence or otherwise, or from any use or operation of any methods, products, instructions or ideas contained in the material herein. Because of rapid advances in the medical sciences, in particular, independent verification of diagnoses and drug dosages should be made.

Although all advertising material is expected to conform to ethical (medical) standards, inclusion in this publication does not constitute a guarantee or endorsement of the quality or value of such product or of the claims made of it by its manufacturer.

Otolaryngologic Clinics of North America (ISSN 0030-6665) is published bimonthly by Elsevier, Inc., 360 Park Avenue South, New York, NY 10010-1710. Months of issue are February, April, June, August, October, and December. Business and Editorial Offices: 1600 John F. Kennedy Blvd., Suite 1800, Philadelphia, PA 19103-2899. Customer Service Office: 6277 Sea Harbor Drive, Orlando, FL 32887-4800. Periodicals postage paid at New York, NY and additional mailing offices. Subscription prices are $424.00 per year (US individuals), $947.00 per year (US institutions), $100.00 per year (US & Canadian student/resident), $548.00 per year (Canadian individuals), $1200.00 per year (Canadian institutions), $592.00 per year (international individuals), $1200.00 per year (international institutions), $270.00 per year (international student/resident). Foreign air speed delivery is included in all *Clinics'* subscription prices. All prices are subject to change without notice. **POSTMASTER:** Send address changes to *Otolaryngologic Clinics of North America*, Elsevier Health Sciences Division, Subscription Customer Service, 3251 Riverport Lane, Maryland Heights, MO 63043. **Telephone: 1-800-654-2452 (U.S. and Canada); 314-447-8871 (outside U.S. and Canada). Fax: 314-447-8029. E-mail: journalscustomerservice-usa@elsevier.com (for print support); journalsonlinesupport-usa@elsevier.com (for online support).**

Reprints. For copies of 100 or more of articles in this publication, please contact the Commercial Reprints Department, Elsevier Inc., 360 Park Avenue South, New York, NY 10010-1710. Tel.: 212-633-3874; Fax: 212-633-3820; E-mail: reprints@elsevier.com.

Otolaryngologic Clinics of North America is also published in Spanish by McGraw-Hill Interamericana Editores S.A., P.O. Box 5-237, 06500 Mexico D.F., Mexico.

Otolaryngologic Clinics of North America is covered in *MEDLINE/PubMed (Index Medicus), Current Contents/Clinical Medicine, Excerpta Medica, BIOSIS, Science Citation Index,* and *ISI/BIOMED.*

Contributors

CONSULTING EDITOR

SUJANA S. CHANDRASEKHAR, MD, FACS, FAAOHNS
Past President, American Academy of Otolaryngology–Head and Neck Surgery,
Secretary-Treasurer, American Otological Society, Partner, ENT & Allergy
Associates, LLP, Clinical Professor, Department of Otolaryngology–Head and
Neck Surgery, Zucker School of Medicine at Hofstra-Northwell, Hempstead, New York;
Clinical Associate Professor, Department of Otolaryngology–Head and Neck Surgery,
Icahn School of Medicine at Mount Sinai, New York, New York

EDITORS

MARIA V. SUURNA, MD, FACS
Director of Sleep Surgery, Assistant Professor, Department of Otolaryngology–Head and
Neck Surgery, Weill Cornell Medicine, New York, New York

OFER JACOBOWITZ, MD, PhD, FAASM
Co-Director of Sleep, ENT and Allergy Associates, New York, New York; Associate
Professor of Otolaryngology, Donald and Barbara Zucker School of Medicine at Hofstra/
Northwell, Hempstead, New York

AUTHORS

MICHAEL AWAD, MD, FRCSC
Division of Sleep Surgery, Department of Otolaryngology–Head and Neck Surgery,
Northwestern University, Evanston, Illinois

YI CAI, MD
Resident Physician, Department of Otolaryngology–Head and Neck Surgery, University of
California, San Francisco, San Francisco, California

ROBSON CAPASSO, MD, FAASM
Chief, Division of Sleep Surgery, Department of Otolaryngology–Head and Neck Surgery,
Stanford University, Stanford, California

JOLIE L. CHANG, MD
Associate Professor and Chief of the Division of Sleep Surgery, Department of
Otolaryngology–Head and Neck Surgery, University of California, San Francisco, San
Francisco, California

KEVIN COUGHLIN, MD
Resident Physician, Department of Otolaryngology–Head and Neck Surgery, The
University of Tennessee Health Science Center, Memphis, Tennessee

GEORGE M. DAVIES, BS
Medical Student Researcher, Department of Otolaryngology–Head and Neck Surgery,
The University of Tennessee Health Science Center, Memphis, Tennessee

REENA DHANDA PATIL, MD
Associate Professor, Department of Otolaryngology–Head and Neck Surgery, University of Cincinnati College of Medicine, Section Chief, Otolaryngology–Head and Neck Surgery, Cincinnati VA Medical Center, Cincinnati, Ohio

EBONE C. EVANS, MD
Resident in Otolaryngology, University of Minnesota, Minneapolis, Minnesota

OLEG FROYMOVICH, MD
Otolaryngology Staff, M Health Fairview, Minneapolis, Minnesota

MARION BOYD GILLESPIE, MD, MSc
Professor and Chair, Department of Otolaryngology–Head and Neck Surgery, The University of Tennessee Health Science Center, Memphis, Tennessee

ANDREW N. GOLDBERG, MD, MS
Boles Professor and Vice Chair, Chief of the Division of Rhinology and Sinus Surgery, Department of Otolaryngology–Head and Neck Surgery, University of California, San Francisco, San Francisco, California

ROBERT HIENSCH, MD
Assistant Professor, Department of Medicine, Division of Pulmonary, Critical Care, and Sleep Medicine, Icahn School of Medicine at Mount Sinai, New York, New York

LEON I. IGEL, MD, FACP, FTOS, DABOM
Assistant Professor of Clinical Medicine, Division of Endocrinology, Diabetes and Metabolism, Comprehensive Weight Control Center, Weill Cornell Medicine, New York, New York

SAMUEL A. MICKELSON, MD, FACS, FABSM
Advanced Ear, Nose & Throat Associates, Atlanta Snoring and Sleep Disorders Institute, Atlanta, Georgia

RYAN PUCCIA, MD
Department of Otolaryngology and Human Communication, Medical College Wisconsin, Milwaukee, Wisconsin

DAVID M. RAPOPORT, MD
Professor, Department of Medicine, Division of Pulmonary, Critical Care, and Sleep Medicine, Icahn School of Medicine at Mount Sinai, New York, New York

KATHLEEN M. SARBER, MD
Assistant Professor, Department of Surgery, F. Edward Hébert School of Medicine, Uniformed Services University of the Health Sciences, Bethesda, Maryland; Chief, Department of Otolaryngology, Eglin Air Force Base, Florida

KATHERINE H. SAUNDERS, MD, DABOM
Assistant Professor of Clinical Medicine, Division of Endocrinology, Diabetes and Metabolism, Comprehensive Weight Control Center, Weill Cornell Medicine, New York, New York

RAVI R. SHAH, MD
Resident Physician, Department of Otorhinolaryngology–Head and Neck Surgery, University of Pennsylvania, Hospital of the University of Pennsylvania, Philadelphia, Pennsylvania

RYAN J. SOOSE, MD
Director, Division of Sleep Surgery, Associate Professor, Department of Otolaryngology, University of Pittsburgh School of Medicine, UPMC Mercy, University of Pittsburgh, Pittsburgh, Pennsylvania

OMOTARA SULYMAN, MD
Resident in Otolaryngology, University of Minnesota, Minneapolis, Minnesota

BEVERLY G. TCHANG, MD, DABOM
Instructor of Medicine, Division of Endocrinology, Diabetes and Metabolism, Comprehensive Weight Control Center, Weill Cornell Medicine, New York, New York

ERICA R. THALER, MD
Professor and Vice Chair for Faculty Affairs, Department of Otorhinolaryngology–Head and Neck Surgery, University of Pennsylvania, Hospital of the University of Pennsylvania, Philadelphia, Pennsylvania

RACHEL WHELAN, MD
Department of Otolaryngology, University of Pittsburgh, Pittsburgh, Pennsylvania

BEVERLY TUCKER WOODSON, MD
Professor and Chief, Division of Sleep Medicine and Sleep Surgery, Department of Otolaryngology and Human Communication, Medical College of Wisconsin, Milwaukee, Wisconsin

KATHLEEN YAREMCHUK, MD, MSA
Clinical Professor of Otolaryngology, Wayne State University School of Medicine, Detroit, Michigan

Contents

> Obstructive sleep apnea (OSA) syndrome is a destructive and insidious entity mostly underdiagnosed and undertreated. It affects not only individuals but the society as a whole. The costs to the populations can be measured not only in morbidity and mortality but also in the financial wellbeing of a society. Financial burden of this disease is staggering. The social fabric of society is also greatly impacted. Physiologic effects of OSA are far reaching. It has been shown that early intervention with treatment of OSA can often prevent and/or reverse many of the negative outcomes associated with this condition.

> Obstructive sleep apnea (OSA) is a multisystem breathing disorder associated with increased morbidity and mortality. Clinical and operative assessment tools improve surgical approaches to treat airway obstruction. The primary sites of anatomic obstruction are at the levels of the nasal, palatal, and hypopharyngeal airway. The literature suggests a relationship between reduced neuromuscular tone and the age-related increase in OSA prevalence for normal-weight adults. Pharyngeal soft tissue collapse due to reduced airway pressure is defined as the critical closing pressure. Respiratory biochemistry homeostasis is an additional factor in maintaining airway patency.

> A wide range of sleep, psychiatric, and medical comorbidities can present with obstructive sleep apnea (OSA), complicating treatment because of intolerance or low adherence to traditional modalities of therapy. Providers must have heightened awareness of how these comorbidities can affect their patients' OSA and work together as a team to optimize health and well-being in this complex population.

OTOLARYNGOLOGIC CLINICS
OF NORTH AMERICA

SERIES OF RELATED INTEREST

Sleep Medicine Clinics
Available at: https://www.sleep.theclinics.com/
Facial Plastic Surgery Clinics
Available at: https://www.facialplastic.theclinics.com/

THE CLINICS ARE AVAILABLE ONLINE!
Access your subscription at:
www.theclinics.com

Foreword

To Sleep, Perchance to Dream

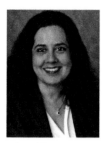

Sujana S. Chandrasekhar, MD, FACS, FAAOHNS
Consulting Editor

Humans have long appreciated the importance of good sleep. Literature and artwork are replete with allusions to sleep, representing rest, dreams, communication with the deity, and death. Poor sleep and sleep apnea are described from ancient times onward.

The link between Charles Dickens and the syndrome that relates to one of his characters was first mentioned in 1918 by William Osler, MD, who noted that "a remarkable phenomenon associated with excessive fat in young persons is an uncontrollable tendency to sleep—like the fat boy in Pickwick" (**Fig. 1**). The Dickensian connection, which was missed or ignored by Auchincloss and colleagues, who first described a typical case, was picked up by Burwell and colleagues in 1956 when they labeled the syndrome Pickwickian. They ascribed the somnolence, cyanosis, polycythemia, alveolar hypoventilation, and right ventricular failure, which characterize the syndrome, to obesity with its attendant increase in the work of breathing.[1]

On the other side of the world, Hindu mythology describes a demon called Kumbhakarna (**Fig. 2**), who had an insatiable appetite and thirst and used to sleep for great lengths of time. He also had an uncontrollable temper. This has been understood in present day to represent hypothalamic obesity and sleep apnea.[2] We, of course, now understand that obstructive sleep apnea can affect people of all body types.

The author F. Scott Fitzgerald very correctly noted that, "It appears that every man's insomnia is as different from his neighbor's as are their daytime hopes and aspirations."[3] Guest Editors Drs Maria Suurna and Ofer Jacobowitz have compiled this excellent issue of *Otolaryngologic Clinics of North America* to reflect the breadth of new and updated knowledge on this complicated subject. Their approach encompasses all current considerations in sleep and looks to the future.

The reader of this issue will find a thorough series of articles on Sleep Apnea here. The authors of each of the articles share pearls of clinical and research-arrived wisdom in the assessment and management of patients with snoring and sleep apnea. It is important that the physician and the patient share goals in the treatment of their

Otolaryngol Clin N Am 53 (2020) xiii–xv
https://doi.org/10.1016/j.otc.2020.03.017
0030-6665/20/© 2020 Published by Elsevier Inc.

oto.theclinics.com

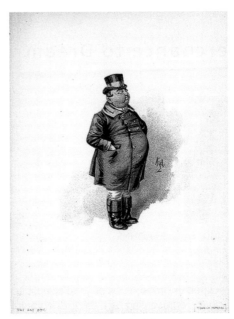

Fig. 1. The fat boy from Charles Dickens, *The Pickwick Papers*, 1889. Character Sketches from Charles Dickens, Portrayed by Kyd (Joseph Clayton Clarke). (Available at: https://commons. wikimedia.org/wiki/File:The_Fat_Boy_1889_Dickens_The_Pickwick_Papers_character_by_ Kyd_(Joseph_Clayton_Clarke).jpg.)

condition. Different phenotypes in sleep apnea need different types of interventions. The patients with other health comorbidities present special challenges. Snoring is quite a common condition; why and when to intervene is an important question. When a patient is sent for a sleep study, it is incumbent on the treating otolaryngologist to know how to interpret the data accurately. Once a diagnosis of sleep apnea is established, the next set of articles look at interventions, both globally with surgical and nonsurgical weight loss, and at all levels of the upper respiratory tract. These can be done at the nose, in the mouth with oral appliances, at the palate and tongue base, both with and without neurostimulator implants, and with skeletal surgery.

Drs Suurna and Jacobowitz preface this issue of *Otolaryngologic Clinics of North America* by writing about personalized treatment of sleep apnea. That is most fitting, as the best outcomes for not only the disorder but also the real and potential secondary health effects are obtained with targeted and individual assessment and care.

Only by doing this can we move from William Shakespeare's equation of sleep with death: *To die, to sleep; To sleep: perchance to dream: ay, there's the rub; For in that sleep of death what dreams may come* (*Hamlet*, Act 3, Scene 1) to John Keats' equation of sleep with rest: *What is more gentle than a wind in summer? ...more soothing than the pretty hummer ... more secret than a nest of nightingales? ... more full of visions than a high romance? What, but thee Sleep? Soft closer of our eyes! Low murmurer of tender lullabies! Light hoverer around our happy pillows! Wreather of poppy buds, and weeping willows! Silent entangler of a beauty's tresses! Most happy listener! when the morning blesses Thee for enlivening all the cheerful eyes That glance so brightly at the new sun-rise* (*Sleep and Poetry*).

I know that the reader will enjoy this up-to-date exploration of Sleep Apnea, guest edited so ably by Drs Suurna and Jacobowitz. The articles will keep you awake, but

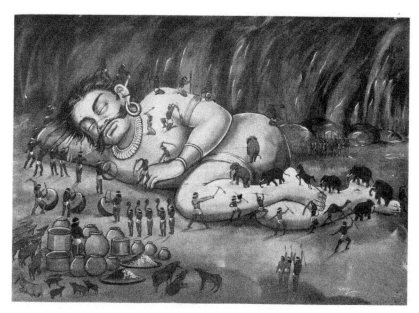

Fig. 2. Kumbhakarna sleeping. (*From* Valmiki's Ramayana, 5th Century BCE. Available at: https://commons.wikimedia.org/wiki/File:Kumbhakarna_wake_up_from_sleep.jpg.)

understanding the subject better once you've read them will undoubtedly help your patients achieve their best sleep.

Sujana S. Chandrasekhar, MD, FACS, FAAOHNS
Consulting Editor, Otolaryngologic Clinics of North America

Past President, American Academy of Otolaryngology-Head and Neck Surgery

Secretary-Treasurer, American Otological Society

Partner, ENT & Allergy Associates LLP
18 East 48th Street, 2nd Floor, New York, NY 10017, USA

Clinical Professor, Department of Otolaryngology-Head and Neck Surgery
Zucker School of Medicine at Hofstra-Northwell, Hempstead, NY, USA

Clinical Associate Professor, Department of Otolaryngology-Head and Neck Surgery
Icahn School of Medicine at Mount Sinai, New York, NY, USA

E-mail address:
ssc@nyotology.com

REFERENCES

1. Vaisrub S. Pickwickian syndrome? The Dickens! JAMA 1978;239(7):645.
2. Lakhani OJ, Lakhani JD. Kumbhakarna: did he suffer from the disorder of the hypothalamus? Indian J Endocrinol Metab 2015;19(3):433–4.
3. Fitzgerald FS. Sleeping and waking. Esquire. December 1934.

Preface

Personalized Treatment of Obstructive Sleep Apnea

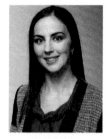 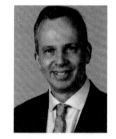

Maria V. Suurna, MD   Ofer Jacobowitz, MD, PhD
Editors

Obstructive sleep apnea (OSA) is both highly prevalent and difficult to effectively treat. Recently, it has been estimated that prevalence of moderate to severe OSA in the United States may be as high as 14.5%.[1] Despite individual and societal burden associated with the disease, OSA remains underdiagnosed, and more importantly, undertreated. The challenge of treatment is related to the heterogeneity of the disease in patients. In this issue of the *Otolaryngologic Clinics of North America*, the contributing authors offer insights to better understand and provide patient-tailored treatment of OSA.

Although positive airway pressure (PAP) is considered the first-line therapy for most adult patients with OSA, only less than 40% of patients utilize it long term.[2] This is not surprising as sleeping while wearing an air-pressure interface is not always accepted nor tolerated by all patients. Patients may be sleepy or nonsleepy, with some symptomatic due to disrupted sleep and others minimally symptomatic, only aware of snoring reported by others.[3] Various comorbidities may affect response and ability to tolerate PAP. Some patients present with nasal obstruction, which causes difficulty with the use of nasal PAP, and nasal treatment, in turn, could improve PAP compliance. The goals of treatment must be considered by the treating physician, as they are vital for adherence to a therapy. Improvement of snoring, daytime sleepiness, and reduction of health risk are all important but do not pertain to all patients with OSA. Matching an effective, acceptable treatment approach to achieve patient's goals is fundamental to successful outcomes.

Upper airway surgery and implantable hypoglossal neurostimulation have a role in treating the large number of patients who do not accept or adhere to PAP or oral appliance therapy. Symptomatic improvement and cardiovascular risk reduction[4] have been demonstrated for upper airway surgery despite the fact that the apnea-hypopnea index often does not normalize. With better understanding of pharyngeal structure and

oto.theclinics.com

mechanics, and by matching individual anatomical features to particular techniques, upper airway surgery has significantly evolved over the last several decades. Thus, particular pharyngeal phenotypes may be better suited for specific pharyngoplasty techniques. However, in cases of severe skeletal narrowing, maxillomandibular advancement may be preferred. The latest and most exciting treatment for OSA is implantable hypoglossal neurostimulation, which carries lower morbidity and does not alter the airway anatomy. Through this less-invasive treatment modality, a collaborative partnership has evolved between surgeons and nonsurgeons. Some patients, who would not seek upper airway surgery, find hypoglossal neurostimulation therapy more acceptable. With increased variety of treatment options and successful outcomes of this new therapy, there is a great potential for improved diagnosis and wider application for all OSA management techniques.

We believe you will find the articles in this issue of the *Otolaryngologic Clinics of North America* both illuminating and practical. Enjoy your readings, and please thank the authors for their work.

Maria V. Suurna, MD
Weill Cornell Medicine
Otolaryngology–Head and Neck Surgery
2315 Broadway, 3rd Floor
New York, NY 10024, USA

Ofer Jacobowitz, MD, PhD
ENT and Allergy Associates
18 East 48th Street, Second Floor
New York, NY 10018, USA

E-mail addresses:
mas9390@med.cornell.edu (M.V. Suurna)
ojacobowitz@entandallergy.com (O. Jacobowitz)

REFERENCES

1. Benjafield AV, Ayas NT, Eastwood PR, et al. Estimation of the global prevalence and burden of obstructive sleep apnoea: a literature-based analysis. Lancet Respir Med 2019;7:687–98.
2. Rotenberg BW, Murariu D, Pang KP. Trends in CPAP adherence over twenty years of data collection: a flattened curve. Otolaryngol Head Neck Surg J 2016;45:43.
3. Keenan BT, Kim J, Singh B, et al. Recognizable clinical subtypes of obstructive sleep apnea across international sleep centers: a cluster analysis. Sleep 2018;41:1–14.
4. Lee HM, Kim HY, Suh JD, et al. Uvulopalatopharyngoplasty reduces the incidence of cardiovascular complications caused by obstructive sleep apnea: results from the National Insurance Service survey 2007-2014. Sleep Med 2018;45:11–6.

The Goals of Treating Obstructive Sleep Apnea

Ebone C. Evans, MD[a], Omotara Sulyman, MD[a], Oleg Froymovich, MD[b],*

KEYWORDS

- Obstructive sleep apnea • Snoring • Apnea hyponea index • Cardiovascular
- Quality of life

KEY POINTS

- Obstructive sleep apnea (OSA) syndrome has significant ramifications.
- Monetary burden associated with untreated OSA as reflected by workplace disability, health care expenses, and transportation safety issues is in the billions of dollars.
- Social and family dysfunction secondary to undiagnosed/untreated OSA has significant negative effect on the social fabric of our country.
- Impact of OSA on human physiology spans across specialties, as it affects neurocognitive, cardiovascular, renal, and metabolic systems.

What are the goals of treating obstructive sleep apnea syndrome (OSAS)? In everyday clinical practice those goals are often reduced to correction of objective markers such as apnea hypopnea index (AHI), oxygen desaturation index (ODI), respiratory disturbance index (RDI), and subjective measures of snoring and Epworth Sleepiness Scale (ESS). Now, one must switch from this narrow perspective to a wide-angle lens in viewing treatment goals. This view opens a global perspective of the burden of OSAS on society. Although obstructive sleep apnea (OSA) refers to diagnosis based on objective laboratory findings, the term OSAS encompasses OSA and a wide spectrum of disease associated sequelae. This wide-angle view of social, economic, and physiologic consequences of untreated OSA ultimately frames goals and end points in the evolution of treatment of this ubiquitous disease estimated to affect almost 1 billion people worldwide.

One must first examine the financial impact of undiagnosed and untreated OSA. The 2003 Wisconsin sleep cohort study, which evaluated the prevalence of sleep apnea in over 3000 middle-aged state employees, found that 24% of men and 9% of women over age 30 had mild-to-severe OSA.[1] From this study, it was extrapolated that the prevalence of untreated sleep-disordered breathing is rising, with at least 12 to 18 million adults in the United States affected.[2] Frost & Sullivan is a growth partnership

[a] University of Minnesota, Minneapolis, MN, USA; [b] M Health Fairview, Minneapolis, MN, USA
* Corresponding author.
E-mail address: froysleep@gmail.com

Otolaryngol Clin N Am 53 (2020) 319–328
https://doi.org/10.1016/j.otc.2020.02.009
0030-6665/20/© 2020 Elsevier Inc. All rights reserved.
oto.theclinics.com

company commissioned by the American Academy of Sleep Medicine to investigate OSA diagnosis, therapy, and its financial impact on the US economy. Frost & Sullivan estimate that there are 23.5 million individuals in the United States with undiagnosed OSA.[3] Given the significant number of adults with OSA, the economic impact of undiagnosed and untreated sleep apnea is too great to be ignored. Untreated OSA contributes to the loss of workplace productivity, increased risk of workplace accidents, increased risk of motor vehicle accidents, and increased health care utilization, all of which places a significant economic burden on patients and society.

In their 2016 report, Frost & Sullivan estimated the loss of workplace productivity to account for 77.4% of the total cost burden of OSA in the United States.[3] This translates to an estimated economic loss of $86.9 billion in 2015.[3] A recent survey of 506 employed US patients with treated OSA found a 40% decline in workplace absences and 17.3% increase in work productivity.[3] Work absences declined by 1.8 days per year.[3] OSA has also been linked to increase workplace disability, which leads to decreased productivity. According to the results of a survey of 150 patients with suspected OSA referred to the University of California San Francisco Sleep Disorder center, OSA is a significant risk factor for work disability.[4] A retrospective pre-/post-claims-based comparison analysis of commercial motor vehicle drivers with OSA, found that the percentage of drivers taking short-term disability decreased by almost 50% in the 2 years following the onset of OSA treatment compared with the year prior to treatment.[5] The study also documented fewer missed workdays in the group receiving treatment for OSA.[5]

Workplace injury or accidents can be very costly for employers, the injured employee, taxpayers, and the entire health care system. Frost & Sullivan found the cost burden of workplace accidents caused by undiagnosed and untreated OSA to be $6.5 billion in 2015.[3] Studies have documented the effect of sleep quantity and sleep quality on workplace safety.[6] Barnes and Wagner found a 5.7% increase in workplace injury when an hour of sleep was lost.[7] As one can imagine, OSA negatively impacts the quantity and quality of sleep, which could increase the risk of workplace injury by affecting vigilance and work performance. In a 2015 study, Hirsh Allen and colleagues[8] found that people with OSA were almost twice as likely to be injured at work. A 10-year retrospective Swedish study by Ulfberg and colleagues[9] revealed that the risk of occupational injury was twofold higher in male patients with OSA and threefold higher is female patients with OSA when compared with the general population.

Individuals with OSA have higher rate of motor vehicle accidents[10] that result in property damage, lost wages, medical expenses, and loss of human life. It has been estimated that drowsy driving causes 328,000 crashes a year, resulting in 1090 injuries and 6400 fatalities.[11] In their 2004 study, Sassani and colleagues[12] attributed 810,000 motor vehicle crashes a year to OSAS. This resulted in 1400 fatalities and a cost of about $15.9 billion.[12] As explained by Sassani and colleagues[12] treating OSA in the United States will cost $3.18 billion but will save $11.1 billion in collision costs and 980 lives annually. A more recent study reported a cost of $26.2 billion in 2015 for all motor vehicle accidents where OSA was a contributing factor.[3]

The health impact of OSA can be costly and catastrophic. Untreated OSA has been found to lead to the development of several serious health conditions that lead to increased health care utilization and significant economic impact. For instance, untreated OSA can lead to coronary artery disease, which leads to stroke and myocardial infarction (MI). In the United States, the cost of treating acute MI was about $14,000 per patient in 2006, and the cost of coronary heart disease was about $190 billion.[13] In 2008, $34.3 billion was spent in the United States to treat strokes.[13] In a patient survey by Frost & Sullivan, diabetic patients who were treating their OSA reported that their number of hospital visits was nearly cut in half.[3] Similarly, Hoffman and colleagues[5] documented decreased health care cost for commercial motor vehicle drivers with treated OSA. In their 2010 retrospective study comparing commercial drivers being treated for OSA with drivers with untreated OSA, Hoffman and colleagues[5] found that the annual health care costs decreased by 37% 1 year after treatment and by 41% in the second year after treatment.

OSA has been shown to have detrimental effects on patient's health and wellbeing. Beyond the negative physiologic effect, OSA negatively impacts the social life of patients and their loved ones. Importantly, OSA should be thought of as a shared social problem that affects the quality of sleep and the relationship of patients and their bed partners. Increased sleep fragmentation, impaired sleep quality, and excessive day time sleepiness have an adverse impact on quality of life of patients with OSA and their bed partners.[14]

The negative impact of OSA on a patient's quality of life has been well documented. In their study of 29 patients with OSA, D'Ambrosio and colleagues[15] reported that OSA impaired all domains of quality of life including emotional functioning, mental health functioning, vitality, and physical health, in the study population when compared with an age-matched normal population. Similarly, several studies have outlined the effect OSA has on a bed partner's quality of life.[16,17] A study conducted in the United Kingdom showed that bed partners had poorer scores on the Short Form 36-item (SF-36) health survey regarding emotional well being, energy/vitality and physical perception such as bodily pain, as well as social functioning. when compared to the normal values for a middle aged UK population.[17] In another study of 37 bed partners, one-half of the bed partners reported being disturbed by snoring every night or almost every night, and one-third reported disharmony in the relationship because of snoring.[18] Patients and their bed partners have reported frustration, exhaustion, interference with work, decreased intimacy, and relationship strain as consequences of sleep apnea.[19]

The main goals of treatment of OSA is to decrease the risk of deleterious health effects and improve quality of sleep. Continuous positive airway pressure (CPAP) is the first-line treatment and most common treatment for OSA. CPAP works by providing positive pressure to stent the upper airway open during sleep, which decreases upper airway collapse and resistance. Several studies have documented improvement in the quality of life of patients and their partners after initiation OSA treatment with CPAP or surgery.[15,19-23] In their 2003 study of 54 patients with OSA and their partners, Parish and Lyng found statistically significant improvement in the ESS and Sleep Apnea Quality of Life Questionnaire (SAQLI) of patients and their partners after treatment with CPAP was begun.[24] The mean ESS decreased from 12.9 plus or minus 4.4 to 7.3 plus or minus 4.0 ($P < .001$) for patients and from 7.4 plus or minus 6.1 to 5.8 plus or minus 4.7 ($P=.02$) for partners.[24] The mean scores on the SAQLI for patients increased from 4.1 plus or minus 1.0 to 4.9 plus or minus 1.2 ($P<.001$), and for the partners the score increased from 4.5 plus or minus 1.3 to 5.1 plus or minus 0.9 ($P=.002$).[24] In a qualitative study by Luyster and colleagues,[19] patients and their partners reported improvement in their sleep with fewer awakenings, decreased daytime tiredness, increase in energy levels that enabled them to engage in social and recreational activities again, resumption of bed sharing, improvement in mood (happier and less irritable), and improved marital quality with CPAP treatment.

The early stage of OSA is characterized as a presymptomatic disease state. Individuals may be asymptomatic or present with minimum symptoms (ie, snoring in the absence any diurnal activity limitations).[25] The body is unable to maintain healthy hemostasis in the presence of long-standing upper airway obstruction. Untreated OSA induces physiologic disturbances such as chronic intermittent hypoxemia, sleep fragmentation, hemodynamic disturbances, and alterations in the sympathetic nervous system.[26] The cellular impact for these disturbances is widespread. Cellular dysfunction ensues by eliciting neurohumoral changes, oxidative stress, inflammation, endothelia dysfunction, and fibrinolytic imbalance.[26] These alterations progress the OSA clinical picture from a presymptomatic disease to clinical disease associated with early onset comorbidities and/or death.

CARDIOVASCULAR
Hypercoagulable State

OSA is linked to specific physiologic systems dysfunction. Chronic intermittent hypoxia leads to increased production of reactive oxygen species (ROS). ROS activates proinflammatory transcription factors producing inflammatory cytokines (ie, interleukin [IL]-6, tumor necrosis factor [TNF] alpha) that induce coagulation cascade. Additionally, inflammatory cytokines impair endothelium function enhancing platelet aggregation through the release of von Willebrand factor and reduction of nitric oxide release. Inflammation also impedes fibrinolysis by decreasing the production of protein C and increasing plasminogen activator inhibitor, ultimately leading to several disruptions in the coagulation counterbalance system.

In Taiwan, a nonrandomized pair-matched cohort study was conducted to investigate the relationship between OSA and the subsequent development of deep venous thrombosis (DVT).[27] Over the course of 4 years, 5680 OSA patients were followed. During follow-up, OSA patients had 3.13-fold increase in incidents of DVT. After adjustment for age, sex, and comorbidities, sex, OSA, and HTN were only factors independently associated with DVT development. Moreover, OSA patients who had CPAP indication had a hazard ratio of 9.575 as compared to OSA patients with no CPAP indication who had a hazard ratio of 2.751, suggesting an increased risk with increased severity of OSA.[27] A 10-year prospective study demonstrated that severe OSA independently increased the odds of fatal and nonfatal cardiovascular events by 2.87-fold and 3.17-fold, respectively. Prevalence of moderate to severe OSA was found to be 65.7% among patients admitted for acute MI. Successful treatment of OSA appears to decrease those cardiovascular risks.[28]

Hypertension

Systems involved in the development of hypertension are the sympathetic nervous system, endothelial function, cardiac function, and renal system. Sleep fragmentation, hypoxemia, and negative intrathoracic pressure activate the sympathetic system. Increase in sympathetic activity leads to vasoconstriction, increased cardiac output, and activation of the renin angiotensin system (RAAS). Vasoconstriction and increased cardiac output independently can increase blood pressure. Activation of the RAAS leads to additional activation of the sympathetic system, water, and NaCl retention, increasing the circulating volume and arteriolar vasoconstriction.

Normotensive moderate-to-severe OSA patients who were not treated with CPAP were found to be 3 times more likely to develop hypertension as compared to patients without OSA.[25] OSA patients compliant with CPAP treatment can benefit from a reduction in diurnal systolic and diastolic blood pressure. The average reduction in systolic blood pressure and diastolic blood pressure is -2.58 mm Hg and -2.01, respectively. The reduction in blood pressure is greater in younger and sleepier patients and those with more severe OSA.[25] Resistant hypertension, blood pressure greater than 140/90 with the use of 3 or more antihypertensives is more prevalent in OSA patients versus those with controlled hypertension, 71% versus 38% respectively.

Arrhythmias

Changes in respiration, autonomic tone, and electrolyte balance disrupt cardiac electrical activity, increasing the likelihood for development of arrythmias. The most common arrhythmia identified in OSA patients is atrial fibrillation. Furthermore, there is also a strong association between OSA and other cardiac arrythmias such as ventricular tachycardia, sinus arrest, atrioventricular conduction blocks, complex ventricular ectopy, and bradycardia.[29] Atrial fibrillation is 4 to 5 times higher in OSA patients, and its incidence increases with the severity of OSA. CPAP-compliant patients have decreased incidence of atrial fibrillation recurrence and a longer control of arrhythmia recurrence off the antiarrhythmic drugs.[29]

Heart Failure and Pulmonary Hypertension

Studies have shown a bidirectional relationship between OSA and heart failure (HF). Despite of patient's compliance with OSA treatment, HF prevalence is up to a 50% in this population.

OSA is commonly associated with increase in pulmonary arterial pressure. This process caused by sleep disordered breathing is referred to as group 3 pulmonary hypertension in the classification of pulmonary hypertension by World Health Organization.

CHRONIC KIDNEY DISEASE

Common mechanisms that propagate renal dysfunction are glomerular pressure overload and hyperfiltration. Untreated OSA is linked to increased renal sympathetic activity, glomerular hyperfiltration, hypertension, and accelerated atherosclerosis. Increased renal sympathetic activity leads to glomerular hyperfiltration. Glomerular overload and hyperfiltration disturb the anatomy of the glomerular kidney subunit by causing glomerular enlargement and sclerosis. A study conducted by Kinebuchi showed that glomerular filtration fraction is higher in OSA patients, and the utilization of CPAP increases renal plasma flow, thereby reducing the filtration fraction.[30] With long-term use of CPAP, the glomerular kidney subunit is less prone to damage, allowing for longer preservation of kidney function.

Several studies have outlined the linkage of OSA to chronic kidney disease (CKD). In patients with CKD and OSA, untreated OSA can lead to accelerated decline in kidney function. A cross-sectional study of 175 patients conducted by Kanbay and colleagues[31] demonstrated decrease in glomerular filtration rate (GFR) as the severity of OSA increased. This correlation held true after adjustment for established risk factors (ie, gender, age, or comorbidities) for kidney disease progression. One of the largest retrospective studies investigating the correlation of OSA and CKD conducted in Tawian demonstrated independent association between OSA and increased incidence of CKD. In a study population of 28,044 patients, OSA patients had a higher risk for developing CKD/ESRD and a lower 5-year CKD/ESRD survival compared with the control population.[32] A third national cohort of approximately 3 million US veterans showed that untreated and treated OSA patients had higher and faster rates of deterioration of kidney function.[33]

NEUROLOGIC
Sequela/CVA

The most studied neurologic ramification of OSA is stroke. Cardiovascular sequelae of OSA such as atrial fibrillation, hypertension, cardiovascular disease, and congestive heart failure can all lead to stroke. Several studies have shown that despite these associated cardiovascular risk factors, OSA independently increases the risk for stroke. An observational cohort study conducted by Yaggi and colleagues showed that after the adjustment for age, sex, race, tobacco use, alcohol consumption, body mass index, and the presence of known stroke-related disorders, OSA maintained a statistically significant association with stroke and death. Furthermore, this study showed increased risk of stroke related death with the increase in severity of OSA, with hazard ratio of 1.75 in mild OSA versus 3.30 in severe OSA.[34]

Neurocognitive

Vigilance and executive function were found to be consistently affected in a metanalysis of 25 studies. Decreased vigilance impedes patients from sustaining attention for long periods of time, which is associated with decrease in work productivity. Changes in executive function can compromise basic skills necessary to adapt to environmental changes. Affected skills may include working memory, planning, organization skills, and problem solving.[35]

Neurocognitive consequences compounded by daytime sleepiness are large contributors to increased motor vehicle collisions (MVCs) in OSA patients. A study conducted by C. George analyzed MVC in OSA patients over a 3-year period before and after CPAP therapy. This study demonstrated that OSA patients had statistically significant increases in car accidents than the control group. Rates of MVC decreased after CPAP intervention in OSA patients, while they remained unchanged in the control population.[36]

Mental Health/Quality of Life

A complex relationship exists between OSA and depression because of the vastly overlapping symptoms. Shared symptoms between OSA and depression are daytime somnolence, fatigue, poor concentration, irritability, psychomotor retardation, and weight gain. Theoretic models that link depression as a comorbidity of OSA attribute the linkage to sleep fragmentation and hypoxemia. Studies have shown that OSA changes the central nervous system structure by decreasing hippocampal volume and inducing white matter changes in the frontal lobes. Neurochemical changes in serotonin, an influencer of the hypoglossal nucleus, also play a significant role in depression.[37] The linkage between this hormonal change and its physiologic relationship between depression and OSA is currently under investigation. Studies analyzing depression in OSA patients demonstrate that the prevalence of depression in OSA patients ranges between 5% and 63%[37] compared with the national average of 6% in the US population.

Quality of life declines in OSA patients because of sleep fragmentation and associated comorbidities. Lower quality of life in OSA patients is associated with increased rates of alcohol and tobacco abuse, use of stimulants, and other substance abuse.

METABOLIC SYNDROME

Increased activation of the sympathetic nervous system in OSA patients has long term deleterious effects on other biological functions. Sympathetic activation promotes gluconeogenesis and insulin release and impairs glucose uptake in skeletal muscles and lipolysis. Long-term activation of these processes can lead to metabolic syndrome. A study conducted at Johns Hopkins found that nondiabetic patients with OSA had a reduction in insulin sensitivity compared with non-OSA participants. Additionally, the insulin insensitivity was directly proportional to the severity of OSA. Patients with an AHI of 15 or greater are 2.3 times more likely to develop diabetes as compared to those with an AHI of less than 5. A study conducted by Steirpoulos and colleagues[38] evaluated baseline levels of high-sensitivity C-reactive protein, homocysteine, total cholesterol, triglycerides, high-density lipoprotein (HDL), and low-density lipoprotein (LDL) in OSA patients and trended their laboratory values over the course of 6 months. Patients who utilized CPAP for 4 hours or greater at night demonstrated a significant decrease in all laboratory values.[38]

PREGNANCY

OSA causes poor outcomes for pregnant patients and their newborns. As gestational age increases, sleep-disordered breathing (SDB) worsens. A meta-analysis of 21 studies demonstrated that the pathophysiologic disturbances associated with SBD can lead to gestational hypertension (HTN), preeclampsia, and diabetes mellitus.[39] Furthermore, OSA in obese pregnant women is associated with increased rates of cesarean delivery (65.4% compared with 32.8%; $P=.003$), preeclampsia (42.3% compared with 16.9%; $P=.005$), and neonatal intensive care unit admission (46.1% compared with 17.8%; $P=.002$).[40]

OBSTRUCTIVE SLEEP APNEA IN CHILDREN

OSA-associated comorbidities expand beyond the adult population. Childhood OSA is associated with cardiovascular, metabolic, and neurocognitive changes. A systematic review conducted by Patinkin and colleagues[41] showed that childhood OSA is linked to the development of dyslipidemia and insulin resistance after controlling for body mass index (BMI). This systematic review further demonstrated increased SBP and higher prevalence of HTN in childhood OSA patients. Neurologic and mood changes that affect childhood OSA patients can disrupt a child's learning ability and lead to decreased school performance. Studies analyzing behavioral outcomes illustrated higher rates of hyperactivity, emotional lability, oppositional behavior, and aggression in childhood OSA patients.[42]

OSAS represents a destructive process, not only on an individual level with its effects on multiple organ systems, but for a society as a whole with heavy social and financial burdens. One should consider wider ramifications of this condition every time one engages in the evaluation and treatment of patients with sleep-disordered breathing. The goals of treating OSAS is to reduce these burdens and keep OSA under control without syndrome related sequela component present. Even though our understanding of this multifactorial disorder continues to evolve and desired outcomes remain a moving target, we should employ all currently evidence based treatment modalities to combat this adversary.

DISCLOSURE

The authors have nothing to disclose.

REFERENCES

1. Young T, Palta M, Dempsey J, et al. The occurrence of sleep-disordered breathing among middle-aged adults. N Engl J Med 1993;328:1230–5.

2. Young T, Palta M, Dempsey J, et al. Burden of sleep apnea: rationale, design, and major findings of the Wisconsin Sleep Cohort study. WMJ 2009;108(5):246.

3. Frost, Sullivan. Hidden health crisis costing America billions. Underdiagnosing and undertreating obstructive sleep apnea draining healthcare system. Darien (IL): American Academy of Sleep Medicine; 2016. Available at: http://www.aasmnet.org/sleep-apnea-economic-impact.aspx.

4. Omachi TA, Claman DM, Blanc PD, et al. Obstructive sleep apnea: a risk factor for work disability. Sleep 2009;32(6):791–8.

5. Hoffman B, Wingenbach DD, Kagey AN, et al. The long-term health plan and disability cost benefit of obstructive sleep apnea treatment in a commercial motor vehicle driver population. J Occup Environ Med 2010;52(5):473–7.

6. Litwiller B, Snyder LA, Taylor WD, et al. The relationship between sleep and work: a meta-analysis. J Appl Psychol 2017;102(4):682.

7. Barnes CM, Wagner DT. Changing to daylight saving time cuts into sleep and increases workplace injuries. J Appl Psychol 2009;94(5):1305.

8. Allen AM, Bansback N, Ayas NT. The effect of OSA on work disability and work-related injuries. Chest 2015;147(5):1422–8.

9. Ulfberg J, Carter N, Edling C. Sleep-disordered breathing and occupational accidents. Scand J Work Environ Health 2000;26(3):237–42.

10. Mulgrew AT, Nasvadi G, Butt A, et al. Risk and severity of motor vehicle crashes in patients with obstructive sleep apnoea/hypopnea. Thorax 2008;63(6):536–41.

11. Tefft BC. Prevalence of motor vehicle crashes involving drowsy drivers, United States, 2009-2013. Washington, DC: AAA Foundation for Traffic Safety; 2014.

12. Sassani A, Findley LJ, Kryger M, et al. Reducing motor-vehicle collisions, costs, and fatalities by treating obstructive sleep apnea syndrome. Sleep 2004;27(3):453–8.

13. Roger VL, Go AS, Lloyd-Jones DM, et al. Heart disease and stroke statistics–2012 update: a report from the American Heart Association. Circulation 2012;125(1):e2–20.

14. Lacasse Y, Godbout C, Sériès F. Health-related quality of life in obstructive sleep apnoea. Eur Respir J 2002;19(3):499–503.

15. D'Ambrosio C, Bowman T, Mohsenin V. Quality of life in patients with obstructive sleep apnea: effect of nasal continuous positive airway pressure – a prospective study. Chest 1999;115(1):123–9.

16. Doherty LS, Kiely JL, Lawless G, et al. Impact of nasal continuous positive airway pressure therapy on the quality of life of bed partners of patients with obstructive sleep apnea syndrome. Chest 2003;124(6):2209–14.

17. McArdle N, Kingshott R, Engleman HM, et al. Partners of patients with sleep apnoea/hypopnoea syndrome: effect of CPAP treatment on sleep quality and quality of life. Thorax 2001;56(7):513–8.

18. Virkkula P, Bachour A, Hytönen M, et al. Patient-and bed partner-reported symptoms, smoking, and nasal resistance in sleep-disordered breathing. Chest 2005;128(4):2176–82.

19. Luyster FS, Dunbar-Jacob J, Aloia MS, et al. Patient and partner experiences with obstructive sleep apnea and CPAP treatment: a qualitative analysis. Behav Sleep Med 2016;14(1):67–84.

20. Siccoli MM, Pepperell JC, Kohler M, et al. Effects of continuous positive airway pressure on quality of life in patients with moderate to severe obstructive sleep apnea: data from a randomized controlled trial. Sleep 2008;31(11):1551–8.

21. Campos-Rodriguez F, Queipo-Corona C, Carmona-Bernal C, et al. Continuous positive airway pressure improves quality of life in women with obstructive sleep apnea. Am J Respir Crit Care Med 2016;194(10):1286–94.

22. Pichel F, Zamarron C, Magan F, et al. Health-related quality of life in patients with obstructive sleep apnea: effects of long-term positive airway pressure treatment. Respir Med 2004;98(10):968–76.

23. Armstrong MWJ, Wallace CL, Marais J. The effect of surgery upon the quality of life in snoring patients and their partners. Clin Otolaryngol 1999;24:510–22.

24. Parish JM, Lyng PJ. Quality of life in bed partners of patients with obstructive sleep apnea or hypopnea after treatment with continuous positive airway pressure. Chest 2003;124(3):942–7.

25. Marin-Oto M, Vicente E, Marin J. Long term management of obstructive sleep apnea and its comorbidities. Multidiscip Respir Med 2019;14(1):21.

26. Kendzerska T, Mollayeva T, Gershon A, et al. Untreated obstructive sleep apnea and the risk for serious long-term adverse outcomes: a systematic review. Sleep Med Rev 2014;18(1):49–59.

27. Chou K, Huang C, Chen Y, et al. Sleep apnea and risk of deep vein thrombosis: a non-randomized, pair-matched cohort study. Am J Med 2012;125(4):374–80.

28. Park JG, Ramar K, Olson EJ. Updates on definition, consequences, and management of obstructive sleep apnea. Mayo Clinic Proc 2011;86(6):549–55.

29. Goyal S. Atrial fibrillation in obstructive sleep apnea. World J Cardiol 2013; 5(6):157.

30. Kinebuchi S, Kazama J, Satoh M, et al. Short-term use of continuous positive airway pressure ameliorates glomerular hyperfiltration in patients with obstructive sleep apnoea syndrome. Clin Sci 2004;107(3):317–22.

31. Kanbay A, Buyukoglan H, Ozdogan N, et al. Obstructive sleep apnea syndrome is related to the progression of chronic kidney disease. Int Urol Nephrol 2011; 44(2):535–9.

32. Lee Y, Hung S, Wang H, et al. Sleep apnea and the risk of chronic kidney disease: a nationwide population-based cohort study. Sleep 2015;38(2):213–21.

33. Molnar M, Lu J, Kalantar-Zadeh K,, et al. Association of incident restless legs syndrome with outcomes in a large cohort of US veterans. J Sleep Res 2016;25(1): 47–56.

34. Shah N, Yaggi H, Concato J, et al. Obstructive sleep apnea as a risk factor for coronary events or cardiovascular death. Sleep Breath 2009;14(2):131–6.

35. Beebe D, Groesz L, Wells C, et al. The neuropsychological effects of obstructive sleep apnea: a meta-analysis of norm-referenced and case-controlled data. Sleep 2003;26(3):298–307.

36. George C. Reduction in motor vehicle collisions following treatment of sleep apnoea with nasal CPAP. Thorax 2001;56(7):508–12.

37. Ejaz SM, Khawaja IS, Bhatia S, et al. Obstructive sleep apnea and depression: a review. Innov Clin Neurosci 2011;8(8):17–25.

38. Steiropoulos P, Tsara V, Nena E, et al. Effect of continuous positive airway pressure treatment on serum cardiovascular risk factors in patients with obstructive sleep apnea-hypopnea syndrome. Chest 2007;132(3):843–51.

39. Pamidi S, Pinto L, Marc I, et al. Maternal sleep-disordered breathing and adverse pregnancy outcomes: a systematic review and metaanalysis. Am J Obstet Gynecol 2014;210(1):52.e1–14.

40. Louis J, Auckley D, Miladinovic B, et al. Perinatal outcomes associated with obstructive sleep apnea in obese pregnant women. Obstet Gynecol 2012; 120(5):1085–92.

41. Patinkin Z, Feinn R,, Santos M. Metabolic consequences of obstructive sleep apnea in adolescents with obesity: a systematic literature review and meta-analysis. Child Obes 2017;13(2):102–10.

42. Rosen C. Increased behavioral morbidity in school-aged children with sleep-disordered breathing: in reply. Pediatrics 2005;116(3):798.

Phenotypes of Obstructive Sleep Apnea

Kevin Coughlin, MD[a], George M. Davies, BS[b],*, Marion Boyd Gillespie, MD, MSc[c]

KEYWORDS

- OSA • Phenotype • Anatomic variables • Neuromuscular integrity • Loop gain
- Collapsibility

KEY POINTS

- Renewed interest in surgical phenotyping of patients with obstructive sleep apnea is a result of a significant rate of poor adherence to medical treatments despite advances in those treatment modalities.
- Disease-related factors contributing to airway obstruction include: (1) anatomic variables; (2) neuromuscular integrity; (3) upper airway collapsibility; and (4) loop gain/arousal state.
- Assessment of patient phenotypes can result in improved surgical planning and treatment outcomes.

INTRODUCTION

The diagnosis and management of sleep-disordered breathing, specifically obstructive sleep apnea (OSA), has continued to grow in otolaryngology. OSA is a complex multisystem breathing disorder, which remains a significant cause of morbidity and mortality worldwide. Although the disorder varies widely in the causes and symptoms of disease, diagnosis and management continue to primarily rely on the patient's apnea-hypopnea index (AHI). When defined as an AHI greater than 5, the prevalence of OSA in the overall population is estimated to be between 9% and 38%, with men affected at a higher rate than women. Another key finding from this study was that 6% to 17% were found to have OSA in the moderate or severe range (AHI $\geq$ 15).[1] Poorly managed or untreated OSA can have a severe impact on patient quality of life and overall life expectancy. Moderate-to-severe OSA is clinically associated with neuropsychological impairment, cardiovascular disease, type 2 diabetes, and sudden death, making OSA a significant public health concern.[2-5] With AHI as the

[a] Department of Otolaryngology–Head and Neck Surgery, University of Tennessee Health Science Center, 910 Madison Avenue, Suite 410, Memphis, TN 38163, USA; [b] Department of Otolaryngology–Head and Neck Surgery, University of Tennessee Health Science Center, 855 Monroe Avenue, Suite 327, Memphis, TN 38163, USA; [c] Department of Otolaryngology–Head and Neck Surgery, University of Tennessee Health Science Center, 910 Madison Avenue, Suite 408, Memphis, TN 38163, USA
* Corresponding author.
E-mail address: gdavies@uthsc.edu

Otolaryngol Clin N Am 53 (2020) 329–338
https://doi.org/10.1016/j.otc.2020.02.010
0030-6665/20/© 2020 Elsevier Inc. All rights reserved.

metric, risk for associated comorbidities increase along with an increased rate of apneic and hypopneic events.

Historically, the mainstay and most efficacious therapy for moderate-to-severe OSA is continuous positive airway pressure (CPAP). The renewed interest in alternative therapies for OSA is, in part, a consequence of poor patient acceptance or adherence to CPAP (**Fig. 1**). With therapy adherence defined somewhat arbitrarily as ≥4 hours per night for ≥70% of nights, the American Thoracic Society has estimated patient adherence to CPAP to be between 46% and 83%.[6] Despite advancement in CPAP devices and interfaces, adherence rates have not improved. Poor mask fit, leaks, xerostomia, claustrophobia, and noise complaints have all contributed to insufficient CPAP use. Loop gain and unstable breathing are additional factors causing poor CPAP response.

Upper airway surgery is an option for this sizable group of symptomatic and/or at-risk patients who cannot tolerate PAP therapy. Because the obstruction in OSA occurs as a result of collapse at various levels of the pharyngeal airway, surgical management requires an investigation into the primary sites of obstruction. Clinical and operative assessment involve assessing body habitus, neuromuscular tone, nasal and oral anatomy, as well as craniofacial structure. Each of these factors may affect the course of OSA and should be considered to choose the optimal therapy. Incorporating patient phenotypes may allow for a more tailored approach to disease intervention and possibly patient outcomes as well.

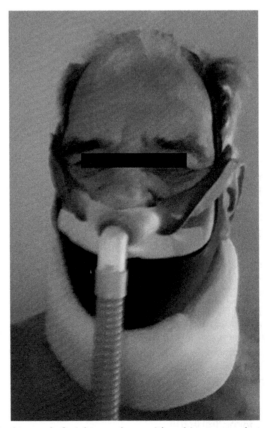

Fig. 1. A patient had to apply facial tape along with a chin strap and neck brace to prevent CPAP leaks.

ANATOMIC VARIABLES

Careful investigation of patient phenotype has remained the cornerstone of planning the surgical approach to OSA. History and physical examinations, polysomnography, airway imaging, and drug-induced sleep endoscopy (DISE) may be used to determine the phenotype. Phenotypic contributions from BMI, neck circumference, tonsil size, nasal airway, and craniofacial structure may result in nasal, palatal, or hypopharyngeal obstruction.

An inadequate nasal airway contributes to upper airway resistance. Nasal pathologies, such as nasal polyps, septal deviation, turbinate hypertrophy, and nasal valve collapse detrimentally alter air flow velocity and resistance. Although this may worsen OSA, nasal obstruction is seldom the sole cause. A 2019 systematic review and meta-analysis noted insufficient evidence that nasal surgery alone is enough to address OSA. Study findings suggest that nasal surgery may improve snoring, sleep quality, and reduce sleep-related arousals but may have minimal effect on AHI.[7] There is significant benefit to surgically addressing nasal obstruction that is known to contribute to OSA and other sleep-related breathing disorders. Decreasing airway resistance can mitigate snoring, improve sleep quality, reduce mouth breathing, reduce nocturnal arousals, and improve CPAP tolerance. Optimizing nasal anatomy with surgery can serve as a primary treatment of mild OSA (AHI 5–15), upper airway resistance syndrome, or as an adjunct in a multilevel surgery for moderate-to-severe OSA.

Tonsillar size assessment is an additional classification tool to categorize pharyngeal obstruction. Adenotonsillar hypertrophy is the primary cause of OSA in the pediatric population, and a less common cause in adults. However, the presence of tonsillar hypertrophy in adults can significantly affect airway patency. Smith and colleagues[8] investigated the effectiveness of tonsillectomy as the sole treatment modality for OSA in adults with tonsillar hypertrophy (3+ or 4+) as the primary site of airway obstruction. This study found a mean AHI reduction from 31.57 to 8.12 in 39 subjects. These findings were consistent within 3 separate BMI groups. In a separate study, Friedman and colleagues[9] demonstrated greater rates of treatment success in patients with 3+ and 4+ tonsils undergoing uvulopalatopharyngoplasty (UPPP) compared with individuals with 1+ and 2+ tonsils.

There is a strong relationship between obesity and OSA. In an observational study, there was a 32% AHI increase with weight gain of $\geq$10% and a 26% AHI decrease with weight loss of $\geq$10%.[10] There are a variety of mechanisms proposed to explain the contribution of obesity to OSA, including its effects on pharyngeal critical closing pressure (P_{crit}). An increase in fat deposition within the parapharyngeal space and base of tongue results in a decrease in luminal volume of the upper airway. Furthermore, neck circumference functions as a marker for regional obesity (>17″ in men and >16″ in women) (**Fig. 2**). Facial computed tomographic scans have been used to observe this concentric narrowing of the retropalatal pharynx with increased volume within the pharyngeal fat pad.[11] In addition, increased abdominal fat reduces diaphragmatic excursion resulting in reduced pulmonary volume. This reduces the inferior traction of the trachea, which improves the tone and reduces the collapsibility of the upper airway. In general, obesity is thought to be adversely related to surgical success. In 2006, Vicente and colleagues[12] observed a negative correlation between the presurgery BMI and change in postsurgery AHI; patients with a BMI greater than 35 kg/m² had less decrease in postsurgical AHI when undergoing a UPPP with tongue-based suspension. This is in contrast to a recent meta-analysis by Lin and colleagues,[13] in which BMI was not found to be a statistically significant factor. Medical weight loss

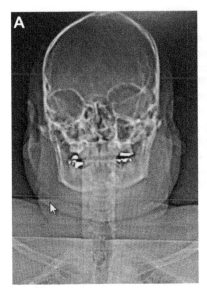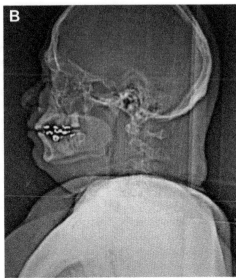

Fig. 2. AP (*A*) and lateral (*B*) neck radiographs of a patient with OSA demonstrating extensive neck adipose tissue loaded onto the craniofacial structure.

therapy or bariatric surgery may be the most appropriate treatment for patients thought to have obesity-driven OSA.[14]

In addition to major maxillofacial anomalies (eg, cleft lip, cleft palate), multiple cephalometric phenotypes are noted as risk factors for OSA. Soft palate thickness and length, posterior maxillary height, malocclusion, tongue length, and position of the hyoid bone relative to various anatomic structures (eg, mentum-hyoid distance) are associated with a higher prevalence in OSA.[15] Cephalometry has been used in an effort to predict OSA treatment outcomes for non-CPAP therapy. Review of the current literature suggests that cephalometric analysis alone is not an effective method to reliably predict treatment outcomes irrespective of the non-CPAP treatment modality, and therefore is not widely applied in preoperative assessment for sleep surgery.[16]

Video examination of the nasopharyngeal airway provides direct assessment of anatomic sites of obstruction throughout the upper airway. Fiberoptic nasal endoscopy is a minimally invasive method for multilevel airway interrogation in the clinical setting. Awake endoscopy has a poor predictive power for assessing postsurgical outcomes but may help to identify associated conditions that contribute to nocturnal upper airway obstruction (eg, nasal polyps, chronic rhinosinusitis, laryngopharyngeal reflux) or tissue hypertrophy, which needs to be addressed as part of the surgical procedure (eg, adenoid hypertrophy, lingual tonsil hypertrophy, mucosal tumors, or polyps). Analysis of palatal, pharyngeal wall, and epiglottic morphology may also be used to direct utilization of particular surgical interventions. DISE classifies obstruction by airway site (soft palate, pharyngeal wall, base of tongue, epiglottis), degree of collapse (none, partial, complete), and pattern of collapse (antero-posterior, lateral, concentric). Although DISE is typically recognized as a more reliable method for characterization of collapse patterns during snoring and apnea events, it has not been established that utilization of DISE results in improved surgical outcomes.[17,18]

UPPER AIRWAY NEUROMUSCULAR INTEGRITY

Neuromuscular integrity is a significant component of upper airway collapsibility. During sleep, pharyngeal muscular tone decreases resulting in a higher propensity for airway collapse. The genioglossus and tensor veli palatini function to maintain airway distention. Mezzanotte and colleagues[19] found that, during wakefulness, patients with OSA displayed higher electromyographic (EMG) activity in both muscles compared with those without OSA, suggesting compensation for insufficient anatomy. At sleep onset, the apneic study subjects showed a profound decrease in muscle activity compared with the control population. With neuromuscular integrity functioning as a protective measure to maintain patency, it has become a growing focus for treatment of OSA.

CPAP adherence remains a challenge for older adult (age $\geq$ 65) patients. The European Respiratory Society published a cohort study observing an age-related decrease in CPAP adherence.[20] Primary sleep disorders, such as OSA, have also shown an increase in prevalence with age. The literature has also demonstrated decreased genioglossus activity measured by EMG with aging.[21] As a result, there is compromise in the protective effect this muscle has on maintaining airway patency. This suggests a correlation between reduced neuromuscular tone and an increased prevalence of OSA with later onset in older, normal-weight individuals (**Table 1**).

Hypoglossal nerve stimulators have been developed to target the neuromuscular mechanism of upper airway collapse. Stimulation of the hypoglossal nerve results in airway dilation in a multilevel fashion, primarily anteriorly. In 2014, in the STAR trial, significant subjective and objective benefit was demonstrated for upper airway stimulation (UAS) in individuals with moderate-to-severe OSA.[22] Increased age may also be an independent factor for treatment success with UAS.[23]

Compromised neuromuscular integrity is difficult to evaluate with routine anatomic assessment. Phenotypic traits of individuals with OSA caused by reduced neuromuscular tone may not be obvious with physical examination alone. Patients of increased age with normal BMI and structural anatomy may have unremarkable appearance on routine head and neck physical examination. DISE may be an important adjunct in this situation to investigate the upper airway during drug-induced sleep in the absence of the airway tone of wakefulness. Reduced tone may also play a role in the cause of positional OSA (POSA). POSA is commonly defined as a 2-fold increase in AHI from the

Table 1
Frequent differences in presentation of obstructive sleep apnea based on age of diagnosis

Factors	Younger OSA Onset	Later OSA Onset
OSA prevalence	Less	More
OSA severity	More	Less
Gender	Male	Equal
BMI	Larger	Smaller
Neck circumference	Larger	Smaller
Tonsil size	Larger	Smaller
OSA effects	CV morbidity; QOL	QOL
Dominant pathophysiology	Tissue hypertrophy; small craniofacial structure	Neuromuscular decline; increased airway collapsibility

Findings are from unpublished data in an ongoing study. *The Effect of Patient Phenotype on Sleep Surgery Outcomes* IRB no. 17-05239-XP.

nonsupine to supine position. Treatments that target tongue and anterior-posterior collapse may be more effective in patients with POSA.[24] Patients with reduced upper airway tone may also have AHI clusters during rapid eye movement (REM) sleep. Grace and colleagues[25] demonstrated cholinergic suppression of genioglossus muscle activity originating at the hypoglossal nerve pool during REM sleep. As a result, treatments that can override this suppressive mechanism (eg, UAS) may serve as a feasible option for this patient phenotype.

UPPER AIRWAY COLLAPSIBILITY

In addition to anatomic factors and neuromuscular control, there may be passive causes of airway collapse in patients with OSA. The upper airway is a muscular tube with minimal skeletal support that exists between the nasal airway and the trachea, both of which have a rigid framework. This flexible structure enables the pharynx to perform vital tasks, such as swallowing, articulation, breathing, and head movements. There are multiple accepted pathophysiological theories of OSA, but the most critical factor is anatomic collapse of the upper airway.

Researchers have used the Starling model to better understand and investigate the forces at work within the airway. In this scheme, the upper airway is the pliable segment between 2 rigid cylinders of fixed diameter and airflow resistance. The pressure at which the upper airway collapses and airflow ceases is the P_{crit}.[26] An inspiratory effort from the lungs generates a negative pressure that gives rise to differing magnitudes of collapse and airflow limitation. Nasal obstruction, P_{crit}, and inspiratory effort all play a role in the airway collapse. P_{crit} is not an easily derived variable and is only elucidated in research sleep laboratories or through mathematical modeling.[27,28] P_{crit} is analogous to the accumulation of soft tissue pressure surrounding the airway, pushing inward.

The more negative the P_{crit}, the more resilient is the airway to obstruction since it requires greater negative pressure to collapse. P_{crit} is typically -5 cm H_2O in normal control patients and is significantly increased in patients with OSA.[26,29] P_{crit} is both sensitive and specific for OSA. This implies that, phenotypically, obstructive sleepers have a fundamentally altered airway, with increased collapsibility being an underlying component to other potential factors. Anatomic characteristics that influence airway collapsibility include mandibular size, hard palate height, and hyoid position, whereas velopharyngeal space and tonsillar hypertrophy are common soft tissue components that compromise the airway patency.[26] Changes to the neuromuscular control of the airway with aging or other insults can increase P_{crit}. Schwartz and colleagues[30] demonstrated that the mechanical forces of the collapsible airway are more impactful of P_{crit} than neuromuscular control. Abdominal obesity decreases lung volume causing reduced downward traction of the airway, which in turn decreases the airway's support from the trachea, resulting in an increase in P_{crit}.[31] Alcohol and other sedating medications affect sleep in a multitude of ways, including an increase in P_{crit}.[32]

Patients with OSA are significantly more likely to suffer from gastroesophageal reflux disease (GERD). Gilani and colleagues[33] performed an extensive database analysis that demonstrated a strong positive independent association between the 2 diseases. Kimoff and colleagues[34] showed that tissues from patients with severe OSA contained significantly more cytokines, inflammatory markers, and oxidative stress than those with mild disease. They also demonstrated greater connective tissue deposition and tissue fibrosis in patients with severe OSA compared with patients with mild OSA. This tissue remodeling can increase pharyngeal wall volume and decrease the lumen size. It can also disturb the muscular responsiveness and force of the pharyngeal muscles to maintain patency.[34] It is debated whether the inflammatory nature of the tissues is a result of mechanical trauma from recurrent vibration and suction, repeated hypoxic insults, or reflux-mediated irritant exposure.[35] Evidence of an association among airway sensory impairment, inflammation, and reflux has been demonstrated in patients with OSA.[35,36] Senior and colleagues[37] demonstrated in a pilot study an improvement in AHI with proton-pump inhibitor therapy and reflux precautions. Despite this small study, it seems that medical therapy for reflux ultimately provides symptomatic improvement instead of AHI reductions. Kim and colleagues[38] showed that patients with concurrent GERD and OSA have worse sleep efficiency and increased fragmentation of sleep, which can improve with treatment of the GERD. These results are consistent with an earlier study that demonstrated significant improvement in sleep quality and daytime symptoms, but no improvement in AHI.[39] More promising results have been demonstrated in children with the use of the leukotriene receptor antagonist montelukast (Singulair) in the treatment of mild to moderate OSA.[40]

VENTILATORY INSTABILITY AND LOOP GAIN

An additional phenotype of patients with OSA is the concept of loop gain within a complex physiologic system that works to maintain a respiratory biochemistry homeostasis. The respiratory system is integrated into a negative feedback loop that is modulated by chemoreceptors, mechanoreceptors, and neural input. The pharyngeal dilating muscles, which work to counteract the collapsing nature of the upper airway, are responsive to blood CO_2 levels, pressures within the airway, and respiratory effort. An increase in the ventilatory drive (normal inspiration) stimulates airway musculature to maintain patency. This respiratory drive increases as flow limitation from a dynamically collapsing airway takes place. This is where loop gain matters, as it is a reaction to respiration challenges. In patients with OSA, as flow limitation occurs from obstruction, ventilation demands are not being met, which amplifies the neuromuscular activity to the pharynx in an attempt to relieve the obstruction. If the airflow limitation is not adequately relieved, an arousal is triggered, and suddenly there is a nonlimited airflow matched with a high ventilatory demand.[26]

A subset of patients have a high loop gain, which is a propensity to unstable respiratory drive. The patients with a high loop gain amplify the respiratory response, which will ultimately lead to an overcorrection and hypocapnia. In turn, this sudden drop in CO_2 levels diminishes the neuromuscular drive to stent the airway open, leading to worsened airway collapse.[26,31,41] These patients enter a repetitive cycle of unstable breathing and obstructions. In contrast, low loop gain does not lead to a hyperventilation reaction, and neuromuscular activity remains stable. Similar to P_{crit}, loop gain is a value traditionally only obtained through research-oriented polysomnograms. There has been some advance into measuring loop gain in the clinical setting with various breath-holding routines, but these have not been standardized.[42]

These cycles, and OSA, are predicated on the arousal threshold (AT). If AT is increased by an intervention (eg, a sedative) in a patient with high loop gain, theoretically the arousals could become less frequent and respiratory perturbations significantly reduced. Accordingly, the neuromuscular activation of the pharyngeal muscles would not be dampened, and overall obstructive events would decrease. In patients with high loop gain, Wellman and colleagues[43] demonstrated that oxygen administration can decrease AHI by half, as well as normalize a loop gain. Oxygen is a known ventilatory stabilizer and blunts peripheral chemoreceptors.

CLINICAL APPLICATION OF PHENOTYPES OF OBSTRUCTIVE SLEEP APNEA

The qualitative measurements of P_{crit}, neuromuscular activity, loop gain, and AT, as discussed above, are difficult and tedious to derive, and primarily done in research sleep studies or via mathematical modeling. Symptoms and polysomnogram can be used to grossly estimate P_{crit}. A high P_{crit} is associated with an AHI greater than 40, CPAP pressures greater than 8 cm H_2O, and predominantly obstructive apneas. Conversely, a low P_{crit} has CPAP pressures less than 8 cm H_2O, and AHI less than 40. A high AT is associated with prolonged obstructive episodes and lower oxygen nadirs. Low AT generally has multiple RERAs, AHI <30, hypopnea:apnea ratio greater than 55%, and oximetry nadirs greater than 82%. Breathing instability is demonstrated by Cheyne-Stokes respirations during sleep, higher likelihood of mixed and central events on polysomnography and nonrapid eye movement dominant pattern.[31,44]

Patients with high P_{crit} (high collapsibility) respond best to CPAP, positional therapy, and weight loss, with an adjunctive or salvage role for surgical interventions and oral appliances. Patients with intermediate increases in P_{crit} (moderate collapsibility) may also have concomitant altered loop gain, neuromuscular impairment, or AT. Therefore, these patients may benefit from anatomic or nonanatomical treatments. Patients with negligible airway collapse with only marginally increased P_{crit} have OSA from nonanatomical reasons, therefore they may be treated with pharmacologic manipulation of loop gain or AT.[31,44]

DISCLOSURE

The authors have nothing to disclose.

REFERENCES

1. Senaratna CV, Perret JL, Lodge CJ, et al. Prevalence of obstructive sleep apnea in the general population: a systematic review. Sleep Med Rev 2017;34:70–81.
2. Kim J, Ko I, Kim D. Association of obstructive sleep apnea with the risk of affective disorders. JAMA Otolaryngol Head Neck Surg 2019. https://doi.org/10.1001/jamaoto.2435.
3. Gilat H, Vinker S, Buda, et al. Obstructive sleep apnea and cardiovascular comorbidities: a large epidemiologic study. Medicine 2014;93(9):e45.
4. Moon K, Punjabi NM, Aurora RN. Obstructive sleep apnea and type 2 diabetes in older adults. Clin Geriatr Med 2015;31(1):139–47, ix.
5. Gami AS, Olson EJ, Shen WK, et al. Obstructive sleep apnea and the risk of sudden cardiac death: a longitudinal study of 10,701 adults. J Am Coll Cardiol 2013; 62(7):610–6.
6. Weaver TE, Grunstein RR. Adherence to continuous positive airway pressure therapy: the challenge to effective treatment. Proc Am Thorac Soc 2008;5(2): 173–8.
7. Sharma S, Wormald JCR, Fishman JM, et al. Rhinological interventions for obstructive sleep apnoea—a systematic review and descriptive meta-analysis. J Laryngol Otol 2019;133:168–76.
8. Smith MM, Peterson E, Yaremchuk KL. The role of tonsillectomy in adults with tonsillar hypertrophy and obstructive sleep apnea. Otolaryngol Head Neck Surg 2017;157(2):331–5.
9. Friedman M, Ibrahim H, Joseph N. Staging of obstructive sleep apnea/hypopnea syndrome: a guide to appropriate treatment. Laryngoscope 2004;114:454–9.

10. Peppard PE, Young T, Palta M, et al. Longitudinal study of moderate weight change and sleep-disordered breathing. JAMA 2000;284(23):3015–21.

11. Jang MS, Kim H, Kim D, et al. Effect of parapharyngeal fat on dynamic obstruction of the upper airway in patients with obstructive sleep apnea. Am J Respir Crit Care Med 2014;190:1318–21.

12. Vicente ED, Marin JM, Carrizo SJ, et al. Tongue-base suspension in conjunction with uvulopalatopharyngoplasty for treatment of severe obstructive sleep apnea: long-term follow-up results. Laryngoscope 2006;116(7):1223–7.

13. Lin H, Friedman M, Chang H, et al. The efficacy of multilevel surgery of the upper airway in adults with obstructive sleep apnea/hypopnea syndrome. Laryngoscope 2008;118. https://doi.org/10.1097/mlg.0b013e31816422ea.

14. Peromaa-Haavisto P, Tuomilehto H, Kössi J, et al. Obstructive sleep apnea: the effect of bariatric surgery after 12 months, a prospective multicenter trial. Sleep Med 2017;35. https://doi.org/10.1016/j.sleep.2016.12.017.

15. Bayat M, Shariati M, Rakhshan V, et al. Cephalometric risk factors of obstructive sleep apnea. Cranio 2016;35:1–6.

16. Denolf PL, Vanderveken OM, Marklud ME, et al. The status of cephalometry in the prediction of non-CPAP treatment outcome in obstructive sleep apnea patients. Sleep Med Rev 2015;27. https://doi.org/10.1016/j.smrv.

17. Certal VF, Pratas R, Guimarães L, et al. Awake examination versus DISE for surgical decision making in patients with OSA: a systematic review. Laryngoscope 2015. https://doi.org/10.1002/lary.25722.

18. Okuno K, Sasao Y, Nohara K, et al. Endoscopy evaluation to predict oral appliance outcomes in obstructive sleep apnoea. Eur Respir J 2016;47. https://doi.org/10.1183/13993003.01088-2015.

19. Mezzanotte WS, Tangel DJ, White DP. Influence of sleep onset on upper-airway muscle activity in apnea patients versus normal controls. Am J Respir Crit Care Med 1996;153(6):1880–7.

20. Martinez-Garcia MA, Valero-Sanchez I, Reyes-Nuñez N, et al. Continuous positive airway pressure adherence declines with age in elderly obstructive sleep apnoea patients. ERJ Open Res 2019;5 [pii:00178-2018].

21. Klawe JJ, Tafil-Klawe M. Age-related response of the genioglossus muscle EMG-activity to hypoxia in humans. J Physiol Pharmacol 2003;54(Suppl 1):14–9.

22. Strollo P, Soose R, Maurer J, et al. Upper-airway stimulation for obstructive sleep apnea. N Engl J Med 2014;370:139–49. https://doi.org/10.1056/NEJMoa1308659.

23. Withrow K, Evans S, Harwick J, et al. Upper airway stimulation response in older adults with moderate to severe obstructive sleep apnea. Otolaryngol Head Neck Surg 2019. https://doi.org/10.1177/0194599819848709.

24. Yalamanchili R, Mack WJ, Kezirian EJ. Drug-induced sleep endoscopy findings in supine vs nonsupine body positions in positional and nonpositional obstructive sleep apnea. JAMA Otolaryngol Head Neck Surg 2018;145(2):159–65.

25. Grace K, Hughes S, Horner R. Identification of the mechanism mediating genioglossus muscle suppression in REM Sleep. Am J Respir Crit Care Med 2012;187. https://doi.org/10.1164/rccm.201209-1654OC.

26. Pham LV, Schwartz AR. The pathogenesis of obstructive sleep apnea. J Thorac Dis 2015;7(8):1358–72.

27. Kirkness JP, Peterson LA, Squier SB, et al. Performance characteristics of upper airway critical collapsing pressure measurements during sleep. Sleep 2011;34(4):459–67.

28. Wei T, Erlacher MA, Gross P, et al. Approach for streamlining measurement of complex physiological phenotypes of upper airway collapsibility. Comput Biol Med 2013;43(5):600–6.
29. Sforza E, Bacon W, Weiss T, et al. Upper airway collapsibility and cephalometric variables in patients with obstructive sleep apnea. Am J Respir Crit Care Med 2000;161:347–52.
30. Schwartz AR, O'Donnell CP, Baron J, et al. The hypotonic upper airway in obstructive sleep apnea, role of structures and neuromuscular activity. Am J Respir Crit Care Med 1998;157:1051–7.
31. Eckert DJ. Phenotypic approaches to obstructive sleep apnoea—new pathways for targeted therapy. Sleep Med Rev 2018;37:45–59.
32. Berry RB, Kouchi K, Bower J, et al. Triazolam in patients with obstructive sleep apnea. Am J Respir Crit Care Med 1995;151:450–4.
33. Gilani S, Quan SF, Pynnonen M, et al. Obstructive sleep apnea and gastroesophageal reflux: a multivariate population-level analysis. Otolaryngol Head Neck Surg 2016;154(2):390–5.
34. Kimoff RJ, Hamid Q, Divangahi M, et al. Increased upper airway cytokines and oxidative stress in severe obstructive sleep apnoea. Eur Respir J 2011;38:89–97.
35. Payne RJ, Kost KM, Frenkiel S, et al. Laryngeal inflammation assessed using the reflux finding score in obstructive sleep apnea. Otolaryngol Head Neck Surg 2006;134(5):836–42.
36. Novakovic D, MacKay S. Adult obstructive sleep apnoea and the larynx. Curr Opin Otolaryngol Head Neck Surg 2015;23(6):464–9.
37. Senior BA, Khan M, Schwimmer C, et al. Gastroesophageal reflux and obstructive sleep apnea. Laryngoscope 2001;111:2144–6.
38. Kim Y, Lee YJ, Park JS, et al. Associations between obstructive sleep apnea severity and endoscopically proven gastroesophageal reflux disease. Sleep Breath 2018;22:85–90.
39. Orr WC, Robert JJT, Houck JR, et al. The effect of acid suppression on upper airway anatomy and obstruction in patients with sleep apnea and gastroesophageal reflux disease. J Clin Sleep Med 2009;5(4):330–4.
40. Kheirandish-Gozal L, Bandla H, Gozal D. Montelukast for children with obstructive sleep apnea: results of a double-blind, randomized, placebo-controlled trial. Ann Am Thorac Soc 2016;13. https://doi.org/10.1513/AnnalsATS.201606-432OC.
41. Pham LV, Schwartz AR, Polotsky VY. Integrating loop gain into the understanding of obstructive sleep apnoea mechanisms. J Physiol 2018;596(17):3819–20.
42. Messineo L, Taranto-Montemurro L, Azarbarzin A, et al. Breath-holding as a means to estimate the loop gain contribution to obstructive sleep apnoea. J Physiol 2018;596(17):4043–56.
43. Wellman A, Malhotra A, Jordan AS, et al. Effect of oxygen in obstructive sleep apnea: role of loop gain. Respir Physiol Neurobiol 2008;162(2):144–51.
44. Bosi M, De Vito A, Kotecha B, et al. Phenotyping the pathophysiology of obstructive sleep apnea using polygraph/polysomnography: a review of the literature. Sleep Breath 2018;22:579–92.

Sleep Apnea Treatment Considerations in Patients with Comorbidities

Reena Dhanda Patil, MD[a,b,]*, Kathleen M. Sarber, MD[c,d,1]

KEYWORDS

- Obstructive sleep apnea comorbidities • Positive airway pressure adherence
- Psychiatric comorbidities

KEY POINTS

- A common comorbid sleep disorder with obstructive sleep apnea (OSA) is insomnia, which should be diagnosed and treated to optimize adherence to therapy for OSA.
- OSA is most common in patients aged 50 to 70 years, a population that frequently has important medical comorbidities that may affect the efficacy of OSA treatment.
- Common psychiatric comorbidities with OSA include depression, posttraumatic stress disorder and anxiety, and often affect OSA treatment tolerance.
- An interdisciplinary team of providers is critical to optimize response to positive airway pressure therapy and improve surgical outcomes in patients with sleep, psychiatric and medical comorbidities.

INTRODUCTION

Patients rarely present with obstructive sleep apnea (OSA) as an isolated medical problem. More commonly, they are hosts to a myriad of complex medical and behavioral health issues comorbid with OSA. The gold standard for treatment of OSA, positive airway pressure (PAP), is highly effective when patients are motivated to use it regularly and as prescribed. However, comorbid sleep, medical and psychiatric disorders can significantly affect usage of PAP, and multiple reports in the literature document overall low compliance with PAP despite its efficacy. An interdisciplinary team consisting of sleep medicine, otolaryngology, dental, neurology, and mental health professionals must be available to proactively identify

[a] Department of Otolaryngology–Head and Neck Surgery, University of Cincinnati College of Medicine, Cincinnati, OH, USA; [b] Otolaryngology–Head and Neck Surgery, Cincinnati VA Medical Center, Cincinnati, OH, USA; [c] Department of Surgery, F. Edward Hébert School of Medicine, Uniformed Services University of the Health Sciences, Bethesda, MD, USA; [d] Department of Otolaryngology, 96th Medical Group, Eglin Air Force Base, FL, USA
[1] Present address: 307 Boatner Rd, Eglin AFB, FL 32542.
* Corresponding author. 231 Albert Sabin Way, Cincinnati, OH 45267-0528.
E-mail address: reenadhanda1@gmail.com

Otolaryngol Clin N Am 53 (2020) 339–349
https://doi.org/10.1016/j.otc.2020.02.001
0030-6665/20/Published by Elsevier Inc.

modifiable, patient-specific factors that influence PAP use, and adjust treatment plans accordingly. Alternative treatments for OSA are increasingly available to address issues with adherence related to comorbidities.

SLEEP COMORBIDITIES
Insomnia

Insomnia is characterized by difficulty initiating or maintaining sleep, which results in significant daytime impairment despite an adequate opportunity to sleep. The prevalence of insomnia, which ranks with OSA among the most common sleep disorders, is cited as approximately 35% in the general population in any given year, with chronic insomnia ranging from 10% to 15%.[1] Insomnia is classified as a primary sleep disorder or a disorder comorbid with another sleep, medical, and/or psychiatric disorder, with comorbid insomnia more prevalent in clinical settings and the general population.[2]

Although comorbid OSA and insomnia (COMISA) was first described in the 1970s, interest in a bidirectional relationship between OSA and insomnia continues to grow. One current model proposes that OSA facilitates the development of insomnia via responses to repeated awakenings, which results in dysfunctional sleep. Insomnia with its sleep fragmentation may then affect upper airway tone, causing collapse typical of sleep-disordered breathing (SDB).[3] Current research supports the association between SDB (including OSA) and insomnia. For example, a 2001 study of patients diagnosed with SDB in a university sleep disorders clinic found that 50% also had insomnia complaints corroborated by polysomnography (PSG) measures showing less total sleep time and sleep efficiency as well as greater sleep latency.[4] A subsequent review in 2009 reported the prevalence of insomnia in patients with OSA as ranging from 42% to 55%.[5]

The symptoms of chronic insomnia most often include fatigue and hyperarousal, whereas the most prominent complaint in patients with OSA is excessive daytime sleepiness (EDS). Patients with COMISA have increased symptoms of both disorders, especially those that overlap, such as neurocognitive and functional impairment, slower reaction times, and psychiatric issues.[6,7] In addition, sleep maintenance insomnia is the most common subtype of insomnia comorbid with OSA, which may be related to repeated awakenings with OSA as well as intolerance to PAP apparatus that is disruptive to continued and restful sleep.[1,3,7]

Research is increasingly dedicated to the common clinical experience that many patients with COMISA experience difficulty adjusting to PAP. Many reports have documented that adherence to PAP is less than ideal in the general sleep population, and some studies show that insomnia further worsens PAP tolerance.[7,8] In 1 study in which 37% of newly diagnosed patients with OSA reported at least 1 insomnia complaint, sleep maintenance insomnia was inversely related to average nightly minutes of PAP usage.[7] It is of significant clinical importance to learn whether patients with OSA also have insomnia before treatment, given their propensity for intolerance to PAP. If insomnia is not discovered through a focused sleep history, an understanding of the most effective options for an individual patient may be limited and potentially result in suboptimal treatment of OSA.[6]

Treatment of COMISA is challenging and often requires intensive counseling of patients to assist them with optimal use of therapy, whether it involves individualized adjustment of PAP for comfort or a careful review of medications that may cause wakefulness or suppress respiratory drive. Sleep medicine providers should access behavioral health resources to provide the best treatment of each separate disorder.

For example, cognitive behavior therapy for insomnia (CBTi) is a highly effective modality of treatment focusing on the patient's maladaptive beliefs and altering the conditioned insomnia response.[6] CBTi has been shown to be more effective in both the short and the long term compared with pharmacotherapy and is often preferred by patients with insomnia.[2,6] Critics of the use of CBTi in patients with COMISA express concern about sleep restriction at the start of therapy that may increase EDS to the point where it may pose unacceptable risk (eg, motor vehicle accident). Despite its efficacy, CBTi may not be an option for many patients given the dearth of professionals trained in this behavioral health treatment modality.[6]

Pharmacotherapy is commonly used to treat insomnia when comorbid with OSA because it is more accessible for patients and clinicians than CBTi. Medications are generally classified as sedatives and/or hypnotics. Benzodiazepines, such as temazepam and triazolam, may be prescribed and also possess anxiolytic properties. Disadvantages include dose-dependent respiratory depression that can worsen OSA as well as rebound insomnia and increased anxiety on withdrawal.[6] Nonbenzodiazepines such as eszopiclone, zolpidem, and zaleplon mediate sedation and amnesia but not anxiolysis. They have less impact on respiratory control mechanisms and have been shown to be of benefit in patients with COMISA.[7]

Rapid Eye Movement Behavior Disorder

Rapid eye movement (REM) behavior disorder (RBD) is a parasomnia whereby patients act out their dreams, often in a violent manner, while muscular tone is paradoxically maintained during REM sleep.[9] RBD can be associated with the presence and/or development of neurodegenerative diseases known as alpha-synucleinopathies (eg, Parkinson disease, multisystem atrophy, and Lewy body dementia), and is often common in narcolepsy.[9,10] Some studies have found that OSA is more common in patients with RBD, and nonmotor symptoms associated with both disorders, including EDS and cognitive decline, can occur in an additive manner when both disorders are present.[9] Adequate screening for RBD should occur at an initial visit to the sleep medicine or otolaryngology service, with questions to bed partners about patients acting out dreams or behaving violently during sleep. If RBD is diagnosed on PSG, a neurologic consultation may be indicated if narcolepsy has been ruled out. Alternative treatments such as surgery or oral appliance may benefit patients who frequently remove PAP masks during abnormal sleep periods in RBD.

Periodic Limb Movement Disorder

A diagnosis of periodic limb movement disorder (PLMD) is based on findings of nocturnal, repetitive movements of the lower extremities at rates of 5 or more per hour of sleep and is often associated with hypersomnia or insomnia. Although evidence is not conclusive, some data show that PLMD may be associated with OSA. In 1 study, PLMD was 3 times more common in the OSA group than in controls and PLMD frequency was associated with the severity of OSA.[11] In addition, limb movements can lead to arousals, resulting in sleep fragmentation and nonrestorative sleep despite PAP. Another study found that restless leg syndrome (RLS), often correlated with PLMD, was associated with insomnia in patients with an apnea-hypopnea index (AHI) greater than or equal to 10.[1] Clinicians caring for patients with OSA should be aware of PSG data consistent with PLMD and ask patients whether they experience symptoms of RLS. If RLS is present, ferritin should be tested and iron supplementation initiated to achieve a serum ferritin level greater than 75 µg/L.[12]

Central Sleep Apnea

Central sleep apnea (CSA) is defined as greater than or equal to 5 central apneas/hypopneas per hour of sleep, with the number of events making up more than 50% of total apnea/hypopnea events for the sleep duration.[13] CSA may arise comorbidly with OSA, or can emerge as a complication of OSA treatment. In addition, CSA may present with Cheyne-Stokes breathing (CSB), which can be seen in patients with heart failure, atrial fibrillation, stroke, and renal disease.

Treatment-emergent central sleep apnea

Treatment-emergent CSA (TECSA) is a controversial diagnosis but seems to be a distinct form of OSA.[14] The central component of a patient's sleep apnea may be rare during diagnostic testing but be worsened with treatment. TECSA not only occurs with PAP treatment but also with dental appliance therapy, soft tissue upper airway surgery, and tracheostomy.[15] Although the pathophysiology is not well understood, it tends to develop in patients with a high loop gain, whereby small respiratory disturbances (hypopneas and apneas) lead to overcorrecting responses such as hyperpneas as well as unstable ventilatory control. TECSA frequently resolves over a period of weeks with successful treatment.[16] However, continuous PAP (CPAP) may not resolve the central apneas, in which case bilevel PAP or adaptive servoventilation becomes necessary to adequately treat TECSA.

Otolaryngologists consulted for surgical evaluation of patients with sleep apnea must know whether TECSA was noted on a previous PAP titration PSG, and whether or not it has resolved with PAP over time. In particular, it should be determined whether the patient has undergone an adequate treatment duration of at least 8 weeks of PAP, at which point the resolution of TECSA or lack thereof will be clear. In the authors' experience, if TECSA resolves with adequate PAP treatment, the patient's sleep apnea can be successfully treated with surgery without concerns that CSA will complicate future treatment. However, if TECSA persists despite several months of CPAP adherence, surgery is unlikely to be considered successful even if the obstructive component of the patient's sleep apnea resolves. At present, literature on this topic is scarce and more investigation is required to understand the role of TECSA in the surgical treatment of OSA.

Central sleep apnea with Cheyne-Stokes breathing

Patients with heart conditions such as congestive heart failure, atrial fibrillation/flutter, ventricular arrhythmias, and those with renal failure or central nervous system disease may present with or develop CSA with CSB in addition to OSA. The presence of a high loop gain and unstable ventilatory drive during sleep is the underlying cause of CSA with CSB, similar to TECSA. However, unlike TECSA, CSA with CSB is unlikely to resolve with treatment of the obstructive component of sleep apnea.[17] Treatment of CSA with CSB fails because of the nature of the primary disease, which potentiates the ventilatory instability. Therefore, although surgery may have a role in treating obstruction in this patient population, an interdisciplinary approach to address the root cause and improve the underlying disease state is critical to treat CSA with CSB.

Central sleep apnea and opioid use

Although opioids are well known to suppress the respiratory drive after acute use, evidence suggests that long-term use may lead to CSA in up to half of patients.[18] Opioids seem to impair both the hypercapnic and hypoxic responses to ventilatory changes, and this impairment is thought to be dose dependent.[19] Opioid use may also induce long obstructive events with significant associated hypoxia. In addition to SDB, chronic opioid use has been shown to decrease quality of sleep by increasing sleep latency and arousals and decreasing REM duration and slow wave sleep.[20]

The most effective management of opioid abuse in patients with OSA is decremental withdrawal of opioids under the supervision of pain management providers. However, neither surgery nor PAP for OSA in active opioid abusers is effective or safe, because relieving the obstruction by either measure can worsen SDB because of an impaired response to lower blood carbon dioxide levels, which further destabilizes ventilatory drive.[17] Therefore, surgical intervention for OSA in patients with suspected or confirmed opioid use or abuse should be delayed until the opioid use is controlled or withdrawn.

PSYCHIATRIC COMORBIDITIES

Patients with OSA frequently have comorbid psychiatric conditions that can affect the severity of symptoms as well as acceptance of treatment. Patients most commonly contend with depression, anxiety, and/or posttraumatic stress disorder (PTSD), which can also coexist with other sleep comorbidities such as insomnia. The sleep medicine community increasingly recognizes the need to screen patients for mental health disorders to ensure patients are receiving thoughtful, interdisciplinary therapy.

Depression

The most common mood disorder associated with OSA is major depressive disorder. Comprehensive reviews report increased rates of depression of 20% to 63% in patients with OSA but use a variety of screening questionnaires to determine diagnosis. When structured clinical interviews are used using Diagnostic and Statistical Manual of Mental Disorders (DSM) III/IV criteria, depressive symptoms concurrent with OSA were reported in between 23% and 34%.[21] In otolaryngology clinics, the prevalence of depression in patients with OSA referred for surgical consideration was 34% compared with 8% in controls when patients were screened with the Beck Depression Inventory (BDI).[22] Suicidal ideation, which is correlated with depression, was noted in 20.5% of a sample of sleep disorder clinic patients with untreated OSA diagnosed by PSG.[23]

With regard to the association between depression and OSA, opinions differ as to whether depression is caused by OSA or is a frequently comorbid mood disorder. One pathophysiologic model describes the role of hypoxemia and sleep fragmentation of OSA that lead to EDS, fatigue, irritability, decreased social interactions, and an inability to participate in activities, which may augment a predisposition toward the cognitive and somatic aspects of depression. Subsequent weight gain associated with depression can then feed back to worsen OSA.[21]

Numerous studies show that effective treatment of OSA can improve depressive symptoms through use of PAP.[21,24–26] For example, 1 study administered the BDI before treatment and after 3 months of PAP. Total BDI scores improved after CPAP, as did cognitive, affective, and somatic symptoms of depression.[21] A study in a military population found significant improvements in depression by the Quick Inventory of Depression Symptomatology as well as improved quality of life (QOL) assessed by the Short-form 36 (SF-36) which measures energy, vitality, and emotional well-being.[26] In addition, 1 report described dramatic resolution of suicidal ideation in a patient with severe OSA and EDS after 4 months of excellent adherence to PAP.[25]

Despite the balance of evidence showing a positive effect of PAP on depression, poor adherence to PAP continues to be common in patients with depression.[27] It is likely that, just as depression is known to negatively affect acceptance to several medical treatments and therapies, it may also directly negatively affect adherence to PAP usage. In addition, depressed patients tend to be more sensitive to perceived impairments and may be less likely to report improvement of EDS and fatigue even if they are compliant with PAP.[27] This patient population will benefit from communication between providers to ensure that depression is being adequately addressed not only to help tolerate PAP but also to optimize a perceived reduction in symptoms of OSA with appropriate treatment.

Posttraumatic Stress Disorder

PTSD is increasingly recognized as a comorbid condition frequently associated with OSA, particularly in military and veteran populations. PTSD is defined by DSM-V as a specific cluster of symptoms, including disturbed sleep, after exposure to a traumatic event that elicits a response of fear, helplessness, and horror. Multiple studies support the relationship between PTSD and OSA whereby frequent arousals and sleep fragmentation during REM sleep in patients with preexisting OSA can prevent recovery from exposure to traumatic events and lead to PTSD.[28] Alternatively, increased arousals and sleep fragmentation related to insomnia, as well as frequent awakenings in PTSD, have been shown to lead to a lower pharyngeal critical closing pressure, increasing the risk of upper airway collapsibility.[29] These data suggest that PTSD and OSA reinforce each other in a bidirectional manner.[28]

Multiple studies of diverse populations with PTSD support subjective and objective associations with sleep disorders, including OSA, upper airway resistance syndrome, insomnia, and nightmares.[4,30] A 2017 meta-analysis found the pooled prevalence rate of OSA was 76% in patients with PTSD with AHI greater than 5, and 44% with AHI greater than 10.[30] Several recent studies support concerns that comorbid PTSD and OSA negatively affect patients, particularly with regard to cognition, QOL, and suicidality.[31,32] Most concerning is the dramatically higher rate of suicidal ideation noted in a study in patients with both PTSD and OSA (51%) compared with those with OSA alone (4%).[32]

A growing body of evidence has shown that successful use of PAP improves PTSD symptoms as well as self-reported sleepiness, energy, and emotional well-being as reported by SF-36 QOL measures.[26,31] However, similar to patients with OSA and depression, those with OSA and PTSD also encounter barriers to effective PAP therapy.[33] Studies of PAP use in active duty military patients and veterans with OSA report that only 25% to 41% of patients with PTSD used PAP regularly compared with 58% to 70% of those without PTSD,[26,33,34] with reported reasons for nonadherence including mask discomfort, claustrophobia, and air hunger.[34] These patients tend to be particularly recalcitrant to traditional therapy and benefit from close mental health follow-up as well as referral to otolaryngology and dental services for alternative treatments.

Anxiety

Another common mental health disorder is anxiety, reported as comorbid with OSA in 11% to 70% of patients.[35] Although it can occur alone with OSA, anxiety frequently coexists with depression and/or PTSD. The benefits of effective treatment of anxiety and OSA with PAP are less clear than with comorbid depression and PTSD, although a review from 2016 showed a moderate impact of PAP on pretreatment and posttreatment anxiety measures.[24] In patients with anxiety, clinicians need to be aware that PAP adherence may be significantly worse in patients who have panic attacks, mask claustrophobia, and other anxiety-related symptoms.

MEDICAL COMORBIDITIES
Craniofacial Disorders

Patients with craniofacial (CF) disorders require special consideration with regard to treatment of OSA. Common CF disorders such as cleft lip and/or palate, Pierre-Robin sequence, craniosynostosis, Down syndrome and other chromosomal/congenital syndromes are associated with a high incidence of OSA. In addition, persistent OSA is more common after adenotonsillectomy in these children than in those without CF disorders. Analysis of drug-induced sleep endoscopy in children and adults with CF disorders shows a high incidence of multilevel obstruction.[36] Therefore, it is important to perform a postoperative sleep study in this population, particularly in children, whose postoperative course is often determined by symptoms. Otolaryngologists should be prepared to treat these patients with multilevel surgery and consider orthognathic surgery to optimize the craniofacial structure. Because other medical comorbidities, such as cardiac and neurologic problems, are common in patients with CF disorders, it is also important to discuss difficult airway and perioperative management with the anesthesia team before surgery.

There is also concern that long-term compression of the midface with a PAP mask may affect facial growth and cause or worsen midface retrusion. Studies examining this potential effect are inconclusive.[36,37] However, the largest study to date found that maxillary retrusion and decreased caudal rotation of the hard palate occurred in children with a CF disorder and OSA that were compliant with PAP therapy compared with a matched group of noncompliant children.[37] This arrest and/or reversal of normal maxillary growth is very concerning in a population that already has a CF deficit present. Although prospective studies are necessary to confirm these findings, an interdisciplinary team with sleep medicine, otolaryngology, dentistry, and oral surgery is necessary to optimize outcomes.

Obesity

Obesity is the chronic disease of our time defined as a body mass index (BMI) greater than 30, with morbid obesity defined as BMI greater than 35. It is a rapidly increasing pandemic, with a current estimated prevalence of 13.6% globally[38] and 39.8% in the United States.[39] Obesity and OSA have a bidirectional direct relationship, with each 1% change in weight resulting in a 3% change in AHI.[40] Studies of morbidly obese patients undergoing bariatric surgery reveal a rate of OSA between 70% and 90%.[41] Obesity is also associated with an inflammatory state and impaired fibrinolysis, and has been shown to be an independent risk factor for venous thromboembolism (VTE), with a relative risk of 2.5 for deep vein thrombosis and 2.2 for pulmonary embolus compared with nonobese controls in a large study of hospitalized patients.[42]

For otolaryngologists, obesity poses several challenges in the perioperative management of patients with OSA. Obesity increases the risk of respiratory compromise after surgery, as has been shown after uvulopalatopharyngoplasty, adenotonsillectomy, and other otolaryngologic surgeries.[43] Preoperative consultation and a close working relationship with the anesthesia team is of the utmost importance in preventing respiratory complications. The risk for VTE must be addressed by the operative team ensuring that patients have sequential compression devices, early ambulation, and potentially anticoagulation in the perioperative period. Ultimately, otolaryngologists must counsel patients that morbid obesity, in particular, decreases the success of any upper airway surgery to ameliorate OSA.

Beyond Positive Airway Pressure

Although PAP continues to be the gold standard for treatment of OSA whether or not the patients have comorbidities such as insomnia or depression, it is evident from the previous discussion that many of these patients do not tolerate PAP. Individualized treatment allows providers to categorize reasons for intolerance or lack of adherence and provide an alternative treatment strategy that may augment or replace PAP.

Oral appliance therapy

The mandibular advancement device (MAD), also referred to in the literature as a mandibular repositioning appliance, is a noninvasive therapy that prevents upper airway collapse by protruding the mandible anteriorly, thus altering the jaw and tongue position. It is most effective for patients with mild to moderate OSA but may not be a viable option for those with poor dentition and/or temporomandibular joint disease.[44] As an alternative to PAP, a recent study in patients with OSA and comorbid PTSD showed that use of the MAD reduced PTSD severity and improved QOL as well as CPAP. In addition, more than half of patients preferred MAD to CPAP. However, 71% of CPAP titrated participants had complete resolution of OSA with CPAP compared with only 14% with MAD.[45] These results show that although MAD may not resolve OSA, it may be an effective adjunct or replacement therapy for patients who cannot use PAP for a variety of reasons.

Upper airway surgery

Surgery affecting the upper airway in an effort to favorably change collapse patterns in OSA include uvulopalatopharyngoplasty, lateral expansion pharyngoplasty, partial midline glossectomy, and hyoid suspension, and offers another option for patients unable to tolerate traditional therapy such as PAP. A 2008 review reported surgical success (defined as 50% improvement from baseline AHI and AHI<20) in 66% of patients undergoing multilevel UAS.[46] Another study found that sleep surgeries affecting the upper airway improve QOL at least as well as PAP.[7] However, pharyngeal surgery can involve significant discomfort and prolonged recovery periods with difficulty controlling results. Experience dictates that surgery often results in partial or temporary improvement and may not preclude need for PAP in the long run, which may signify limited benefit for upper airway surgery in patients with comorbidities severe enough to preclude PAP use.

Hypoglossal nerve stimulation

A promising surgical alternative for patients unable to tolerate PAP is the hypoglossal nerve stimulator (HNS), which was approved in the United States in 2014 for use in select patients who meet candidacy. This fully implantable device produces protrusion and stiffening of the tongue during each inspiration to reduce upper airway collapse and improve airflow during sleep. The HNS has been shown to improve OSA severity and daytime sleepiness in premarket and postmarket studies and is well tolerated by patients.[47] The device may be particularly suitable for patients with craniofacial anomalies who cannot be fitted with a mask for PAP as well as for patients with insomnia, PTSD and anxiety, and who are sensitized to the presence of a mask for reasons such as claustrophobia, combat trauma, and simple discomfort. However, it is important to remember that, similar to PAP, HNS is a patient-controlled device. Despite the proven efficacy of HNS, patients with poor previous adherence to PAP caused by comorbid sleep and psychiatric conditions may have similar obstacles to use of HNS, highlighting the need to counsel patients preoperatively to ensure receptivity to the device after surgery.

SUMMARY

A wide range of comorbid sleep, psychiatric, and medical comorbidities can present with OSA, complicating treatment because of poor adherence to or lack of efficacy of traditional modalities of therapy such as PAP. Providers must have a heightened awareness of how these comorbidities can affect their patients' OSA and work as a team to optimize health and well-being in this complex population.

DISCLOSURE

The authors have nothing to disclose.

REFERENCES

1. Krell SB, Kapur VK. Insomnia complaints in patients evaluated for obstructive sleep apnea. Sleep Breath 2005;9(3):104–10.
2. Edinger JD, Olsen MK, Stechuchak KM, et al. Cognitive behavioral therapy for patients with primary insomnia or insomnia associated predominantly with mixed psychiatric disorders: a randomized clinical trial. Sleep 2009;32(4):499–510.
3. Zhang Y, Ren R, Lei F, et al. Worldwide and regional prevalence rates of co-occurrence of insomnia and insomnia symptoms with obstructive sleep apnea: a systematic review and meta-analysis. Sleep Med Rev 2019;45:1–17.
4. Krakow B, Melendrez D, Ferreira E, et al. Prevalence of insomnia symptoms in patients with sleep-disordered breathing. Chest 2001;120(6):1923–9.
5. Benetó A, Gomez-Siurana E, Rubio-Sanchez P. Comorbidity between sleep apnea and insomnia. Sleep Med Rev 2009;13(4):287–93.
6. Lack L, Sweetman A. Diagnosis and treatment of insomnia comorbid with obstructive sleep apnea. Sleep Med Clin 2016;11(3):379–88.
7. Wickwire EM, Smith MT, Birnbaum S, et al. Sleep maintenance insomnia complaints predict poor CPAP adherence: A clinical case series. Sleep Med 2010; 11(8):772–6.
8. Pieh C, Bach M, Popp R, et al. Insomnia symptoms influence CPAP compliance. Sleep Breath 2013;17(1):99–104.
9. Bugalho P, Mendonça M, Barbosa R, et al. The influence of sleep disordered breathing in REM sleep behavior disorder. Sleep Med 2017;37:210–5.
10. Zhang J, Li SX, Lam SP, et al. REM sleep behavior disorder and obstructive sleep apnea: does one "evil" make the other less or more "evil"? Sleep Med 2017;37: 216–7.
11. Yalın OÖ, Yılmaz İA, Sungur MA, et al. Obstructive sleep apnea syndrome, periodic limb movements and related factors. Turk J Neurol 2015;21:90–4.
12. Allen RP, Picchietti DL, Auerbach M, et al. Evidence-based and consensus clinical practice guidelines for the iron treatment of restless legs syndrome/Willis-Ekbom disease in adults and children: an IRLSSG task force report. Sleep Med 2018;41:27–44.
13. American Academy of Sleep Medicine. International classification of sleep disorders. Darien (IL): American Academy of Sleep Medicine; 2014.
14. Wang J, Wang Y, Feng J, et al. Complex sleep apnea syndrome. Patient Prefer Adherence 2013;7:633–41.
15. Goldstein C, Kuzniar TJ. The emergence of central sleep apnea after surgical relief of nasal obstruction in obstructive sleep apnea. J Clin Sleep Med 2012;8(3): 321–2.

16. Dernaika T, Tawk M, Nazir S, et al. The significance and outcome of continuous positive airway pressure-related central sleep apnea during split-night sleep studies. Chest 2007;132(1):81–7.

17. Kryger MH, Roth T. Principles and practice of sleep medicine. 6th edition. Philadelphia: Elsevier; 2017.

18. Wang D, Teichtahl H, Drummer O, et al. Central sleep apnea in stable methadone maintenance treatment patients. Chest 2005;128(3):1348–56.

19. Weil JV, McCullough RE, Kline JS, et al. Diminished ventilatory response to hypoxia and hypercapnia after morphine in normal man. N Engl J Med 1975;292(21):1103–6.

20. Hartwell EE, Pfeifer JG, McCauley JL, et al. Sleep disturbances and pain among individuals with prescription opioid dependence. Addict Behav 2014;39(10):1537–42.

21. Means MK, Lichstein KL, Edinger JD, et al. Changes in depressive symptoms after continuous positive airway pressure treatment for obstructive sleep apnea. Sleep Breath 2003;7(1):31–42.

22. Ishman SL, Cavey RM, Mettel TL, et al. Depression, sleepiness, and disease severity in patients with obstructive sleep apnea. Laryngoscope 2010;120(11):2331–5.

23. Choi SJ, Joo EY, Lee YJ, et al. Suicidal ideation and insomnia symptoms in subjects with obstructive sleep apnea syndrome. Sleep Med 2015;16(9):1146–50.

24. Gupta MA, Simpson FC, Lyons DCA. The effect of treating obstructive sleep apnea with positive airway pressure on depression and other subjective symptoms: A systematic review and meta-analysis. Sleep Med Rev 2016;28:55–68.

25. Krahn LE, Miller BW, Bergstrom LR. Rapid resolution of intense suicidal ideation after treatment of severe obstructive sleep apnea. J Clin Sleep Med 2008;4(1):64–5.

26. Mysliwiec V, Capaldi VF, Gill J, et al. Adherence to positive airway pressure therapy in US military personnel with sleep apnea improves sleepiness, sleep quality, and depressive symptoms. Mil Med 2015;180(4):475–82.

27. Wells RD, Freedland KE, Carney RM, et al. Adherence, reports of benefits, and depression among patients treated with continuous positive airway pressure. Psychosom Med 2007;69(5):449–54.

28. Jaoude P, Vermont LN, Porhomayon J, et al. Sleep-disordered breathing in patients with post-traumatic stress disorder. Ann Am Thorac Soc 2015;12(2):259–68.

29. Sériès F, Roy N, Marc I. Effects of sleep deprivation and sleep fragmentation on upper airway collapsibility in normal subjects. Am J Respir Crit Care Med 1994;150(2):481–5.

30. Zhang Y, Weed JG, Ren R, et al. Prevalence of obstructive sleep apnea in patients with posttraumatic stress disorder and its impact on adherence to continuous positive airway pressure therapy: a meta-analysis. Sleep Med 2017;36:125–32.

31. Lettieri CJ, Williams SG, Collen JF. OSA syndrome and posttraumatic stress disorder: clinical outcomes and impact of positive airway pressure therapy. Chest 2016;149(2):483–90.

32. Magruder KM, Christopher Frueh B, Knapp RG, et al. Prevalence of posttraumatic stress disorder in Veterans Affairs primary care clinics. Gen Hosp Psychiatry 2005;27(3):169–79.

33. Collen JF, Lettieri CJ, Hoffman M. The impact of posttraumatic stress disorder on CPAP adherence in patients with obstructive sleep apnea. J Clin Sleep Med 2012;8(6):667–72.
34. El-Solh AA, Ayyar L, Akinnusi M, et al. Positive airway pressure adherence in veterans with posttraumatic stress disorder. Sleep 2010;33(11):1495–500.
35. Saunamäki T, Jehkonen M. Depression and anxiety in obstructive sleep apnea syndrome: a review. Acta Neurol Scand 2007;116(5):277–88.
36. Korayem MM, Witmans M, MacLean J, et al. Craniofacial morphology in pediatric patients with persistent obstructive sleep apnea with or without positive airway pressure therapy: a cross-sectional cephalometric comparison with controls. Am J Orthod Dentofacial Orthop 2013;144(1):78–85.
37. Roberts SD, Kapadia H, Greenlee G, et al. Midfacial and dental changes associated with nasal positive airway pressure in children with obstructive sleep apnea and craniofacial conditions. J Clin Sleep Med 2016;12(4):469–75.
38. Prevalence of obesity among adults, BMI ≥30, age-standardized - Estimates by WHO region. Available at: http://apps.who.int/gho/data/view.main.REGION 2480A?lang=en. Accessed September 14, 2019.
39. Adult Obesity Facts | Overweight & Obesity | CDC. 2019. Available at: https://www.cdc.gov/obesity/data/adult.html. Accessed September 27, 2019.
40. Peppard PE, Young T, Palta M, et al. Longitudinal study of moderate weight change and sleep-disordered breathing. JAMA 2000;284(23):3015–21.
41. Ortiz VE, Kwo J. Obesity: physiologic changes and implications for preoperative management. BMC Anesthesiol 2015;15:97.
42. Stein PD, Beemath A, Olson RE. Obesity as a risk factor in venous thromboembolism. Am J Med 2005;118(9):978–80.
43. Doyle SL, Lysaght J, Reynolds JV. Obesity and post-operative complications in patients undergoing non-bariatric surgery. Obes Rev 2010;11(12):875–86.
44. Marklund M, Franklin KA. Long-term effects of mandibular repositioning appliances on symptoms of sleep apnoea. J Sleep Res 2007;16(4):414–20.
45. El-Solh AA, Homish GG, Ditursi G, et al. A randomized crossover trial evaluating continuous positive airway pressure versus mandibular advancement device on health outcomes in veterans with posttraumatic stress disorder. J Clin Sleep Med 2017;13(11):1327–35.
46. Lin H-C, Friedman M, Chang H-W, et al. The efficacy of multilevel surgery of the upper airway in adults with obstructive sleep apnea/hypopnea syndrome. Laryngoscope 2008;118(5):902–8.
47. Certal VF, Zaghi S, Riaz M, et al. Hypoglossal nerve stimulation in the treatment of obstructive sleep apnea: a systematic review and meta-analysis. Laryngoscope 2015;125(5):1254–64.

Why and When to Treat Snoring

Kathleen Yaremchuk, MD, MSA

KEYWORDS

- Snoring • Positional therapy • Airway resistance • Sound intensity • Oral appliances
- Complementary • Alternative medicines

KEY POINTS

- Snoring is noisy or disruptive breathing and is on the continuum of sleep-disordered breathing, and can be characterized as heavy breathing, simple snoring, upper airway resistance syndrome, and obstructive sleep apnea (OSA).
- Not everyone who snores has OSA and not everyone with OSA snores. For this reason, it is vitally important to rule out the diagnosis of OSA in a snorer presenting for treatment.
- Recognizing the difference between OSA and snoring is impossible without a sleep study. The usual history, physical examination, and assessment of hypersomnolence are important for any patient being seen for snoring.
- A diagnosis of "simple snoring" can only be made when OSA has been ruled out.

It is estimated that half of the adult population older than 60 years snores. The many aspects of snoring are discussed herein, including impacts on bed partners, the individual who snores, and when and how to appropriately evaluate, diagnose, and treat the perpetrator of the noise. The goal of this article is to expand clinicians' knowledge base regarding the phenomenon of snoring.

Although many medical conditions are discussed at family gatherings, the mention of snoring and its treatments will often cause the room to go silent momentarily and then burst into activity as family members jump at the chance to tell stories of heroic snoring that rattles the rafters. This usually occurs at the expense of the embarrassed "snorer."

The definition of snoring in the Merriam-Webster Dictionary is "to breathe during sleep with a rough hoarse noise due to vibration of the soft palate."[1] The First Oxford Dictionary in 1911 describes it as making "hoarse rattling or grunting noises in breathing esp. during sleep; bring oneself awake, into a nightmare."[2] Descriptions of snoring go back into the fifteenth century. In different languages and cultures, snoring is represented differently. Many are familiar with "zzz" being the onomatopoeic representation of snoring. The origin of "zzz" to represent snoring is a relatively recent invention,

Department of Otolaryngology/Head and Neck Surgery, Henry Ford Hospital, 2799 West Grand Boulevard, Detroit, MI 48202, USA
E-mail address: kyaremc1@hfhs.org

Otolaryngol Clin N Am 53 (2020) 351–365
https://doi.org/10.1016/j.otc.2020.02.011
0030-6665/20/© 2020 Elsevier Inc. All rights reserved.

having come into common use with the advent of comic strips. The only way to appropriately represent a sleeping individual versus a deceased one was to add the "zzz"s.[3]

Snoring is noisy or disruptive breathing and is on the continuum of sleep-disordered breathing, and may be characterized as heavy breathing, simple snoring, upper airway resistance syndrome (UARS), and obstructive sleep apnea (OSA). Not everyone who snores has OSA and not everyone with OSA snores. For this reason, it is vitally important to rule out the diagnosis of OSA in a snorer presenting for treatment. Recognizing the difference between OSA and snoring is impossible without a sleep study. The usual history, physical examination, and assessment of hypersomnolence are important for any patient who is being seen for snoring. A diagnosis of "simple snoring" can only be made when OSA has been ruled out.

WHAT CAUSES SNORING AND WHERE DOES THE SOUND COME FROM?

Snoring occurs during inspiration, and can rarely persist during expiration, as a result of resistance within the upper aerodigestive tract during sleep. A mathematical model for snoring represents air flow through an elastic or collapsible tube, which is the upper airway[4] **(Fig. 1)**. The collapse of the upper airway in OSA patients is greater when they are asleep as well as awake. Not uncommonly, families will complain that the patient snores when he or she is awake.

As the upper airway narrows, resistance increases, vibrations occur, and sound is produced. Vibration can be generated at the level of the soft palate, base of tongue, or epiglottis. Variations in muscle tone and airway dimensions that occur from nasal or oral breathing contribute to the complex mathematical model.

Compared with nonsnorers, snorers generate more negative inspiratory pressures and prolonged inspiratory time, and demonstrate limitation of respiratory flow. These changes lead to unstable, turbulent airflow and vibration, causing noise production. Because the pattern is unstable, the volume and nature of the noise is irregular and there is difficulty for a listener (bed partner) to habituate to the sound (noise). One needs to remember that the definition of "noise" depends on the listener. Think of

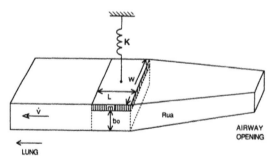

Fig. 1. Upper airways. A collapsible segment is represented as a section of length L with a cross-section approximated as a rectangle of width W (ie, lateral diameter) and depth b* (ie, AP diameter). The moveable wall of the collapsible segment is assumed to have a mass m and to be supported by a linear spring with a Hooke spring constant K; the spring's neutral position is when b* = b. It is further assumed that the moving wall of the collapsible section maintains its parallel orientation with respect to the opposing wall at all times. A constant mean V is assumed in the inspiratory direction. The upper airways, from the collapsible section to the airway opening, are assumed to have a linear flow resistance (Rua). (*From* Gavriely N, Jensen O. Theory and measurement of snores. J App Physiol. 1993;74:2828–37; with permission.)

different tastes in music from classical to heavy metal as being similar in terms of describing "snoring noise" for some bed partners. It is reasonable to ask a patient to bring a recording of their snoring for evaluation by someone other than the bed partner.

In some instances, the difference between noisy breathing and snoring may depend on the listener. Bed partners with low arousal thresholds or very good hearing may find any noise intrusive and disruptive to their sleep. Snoring can be described in terms of frequency and volume or decibels (dB). Another important description is the nature of the sound in terms of regularity and predictability.

White noise is a random signal having equal intensity at different frequencies, giving it a constant power spectral density[5] (**Fig. 2**). Because white noise does not vary in tonality, frequency, and/or volume, it is often considered soothing and is used to block out intermittent noise and lull individuals to sleep. This phenomenon can often be seen on airplanes with sedentary passengers awaiting takeoff of the plane. The continuous hum of the engines is an example of a constant sound that is not disruptive. Snoring, on the other hand, is irregular in frequency and volume. The diagnosis of "simple snoring" is given to an individual when UARS and OSA have been eliminated as a diagnosis based on a polysomnogram or home sleep study.

SOUND CHARACTERISTICS OF SNORING

There is a fair amount of literature describing snoring and its relationship with OSA. There is general agreement that individuals who snore are more likely to suffer from OSA than those who do not. It is also more likely that loudness of the snoring is correlated with the severity of OSA. Maimon and Hanly[6] evaluated 1643 habitual snorers for evaluation of sleep apnea with objective measurement of snoring intensity. The degree of OSA was graded as no OSA (apnea-hypopnea index [AHI]<5), mild (AHI 5–15), moderate (AHI 15–30), and severe (AHI>30). Snoring was measured on a digital sound meter and the mean maximum dB level to classify snoring as mild (40–50 dB), moderate (50–60 dB), or severe (>60 dB) (**Table 1**). There was a significant correlation between severity of OSA and snoring intensity (**Fig. 3**).[6]

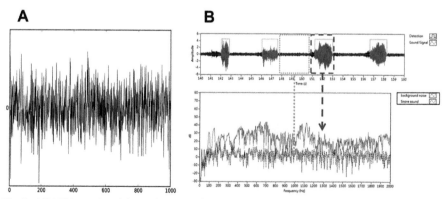

Fig. 2. (*A*) White noise. (*B*) Snoring sound measurements. (*From* [A] Morn. White noise.svg. Available at: https://commons.wikimedia.org/w/index.php?curid=24084756. Accessed October 1, 2019; and [B] Lee L-A, Yu J-F, Lo Y-L, et al. Energy types of snoring sounds in patients with obstructive sleep apnea syndrome: a preliminary observation. PLoS One. 2012;7(12):e53481.)

Table 1
Snoring measurement on digital sound meter

	All Patients	Male	Female
Total sleep time	52.0 ± 6.5	54.1 ± 6.4	47.4 ± 4[a]
NREM sleep	52.2 ± 6.7	54.4 ± 6.5	47.6 ± 4.2[a]
REM sleep	50.5 ± 6.1	52.3 ± 6	46.4 ± 3.9[a]
Supine	53.4 ± 6.7	55.4 ± 6.5	48.7 ± 4.7[a]
Nonsupine	50.9 ± 6.6	52.8 ± 6.6	46.7 ± 4[a]
BMI <30 kg/m^2	49.5 ± 5.3	51.6 ± 5.4	46.6 ± 3.4[a]
BMI ≥30 kg/m^2	54.8 ± 6.7	56.1 ± 6.4	49.3 ± 4.6[a]
Neck circumference <40 cm	49.5 ± 5.2	51.7 ± 5.3	46.6 ± 3.5[a]
Neck circumference ≥40 cm	54.9 ± 6.8	55.9 ± 6.6	49.4 ± 4.9[a]

[a] $P<.001$ versus male.
From Maimon N, Hanley PJ. Does snoring intensity correlate with the severity of obstructive sleep apnea? J Clin Med. 2010;6(5):477; with permission.

As otolaryngologists, sound is usually described in terms of frequency and volume (dB). During standardized polysomnography, there is a lack of standardization for measuring snoring sounds.[7] Snoring reports that are included from diagnostic polysomnography may describe snoring, in addition to usual sleep parameters, but the description of snoring is based on a technician's subjective evaluation and not on objective sound measurement data from a noise exposure analyzer. For this reason, the description of snoring varies depending on whether one is being exposed to it as one is trying to sleep, evaluating a sound meter graph depiction of volume and frequency, or as a technician monitoring an individual sleep pattern during polysomnography.

A study of 1139 patients underwent acoustic measurement of snoring sound intensity during polysomnographic testing.[8] Four decibel levels were measured during sleep using the A-weighted scale that reflects the hearing spectrum of the human ear. The recording microphone was suspended 24 inches above the patient, which should be the distance from a bed partner and would represent the snoring volume

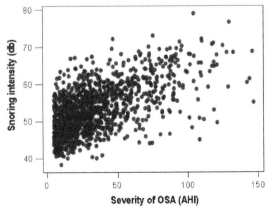

Fig. 3. Correlation between severity of OSA as indicated by AHI and snoring intensity measured in dB. (*From* Maimon N, Hanley PJ. Does snoring intensity correlate with the severity of obstructive sleep apnea? J Clin Med. 2010;6(5):477; with permission.)

they would experience. The patients were positioned in the supine position with the usual polysomnographic monitoring.

An L_{10} value of 40 dBA was exceeded by 78.7% of patients and 50 dBA was exceeded by 34.4% of patients. A Leq value of 38 dBA was exceeded by 84.7% of the patients. L_{10} indicates that for 10% of the recording time the specified dB was exceeded, and Leq is a measure of the sound pressure level over the test period. For patients with a chief complaint of breathing cessation, 48% had a Leq between 50 and 70 dBA. Body mass index (BMI; kg/m^2) and gender were found to be have significant correlation. Men were significantly louder snorers than women. Higher BMI was found to be significantly correlated with snoring volume after controlling for gender at all sound level measurements ($P<.001$). There was no correlation between snoring intensity and age. Snoring sound levels were found to be significantly higher in apneic snorers than in nonapneic snorers even after controlling for gender, age, and BMI. The Leq, L_1, L_5, and L_{10} were 5 dB louder in the apneic snorers.

WHERE DOES SNORING ORIGINATE?

Snoring is a result of resistance caused by areas of collapse within the upper airway. Snoring frequency analysis has been shown to be specific to palate, tongue, tonsils, and epiglottis.[9] Snoring of 16 subjects was digitally recorded during natural and drug-induced sleep endoscopy (DISE). Palatal snoring had a median peak frequency at 137 Hz, Tongue base snoring 1243 Hz, palate with tongue 190 Hz, and epiglottic snores 490 Hz (**Fig. 4**). The site of vibration during DISE was found to have a higher frequency component of sound, which would implicate collapse of the tongue base.

Herzog and colleagues[10] evaluated 60 male patients with possible OSA and snoring. The patients underwent clinical examinations and polysomnography with parallel digitally recorded snoring. The periodicity of snoring was classified into rhythmic and nonrhythmic snoring. Snoring patients revealed peak intensity frequency between 100 and 300 Hz (palatal) and had rhythmic snoring, whereas patients with OSA had peak intensity frequency higher than 1000 Hz and nonrhythmic snoring. BMI correlated with peak intensity of the power spectrum. None of the clinical examination parameters correlated with peak frequency or intensity.

APPS FOR SNORING

In the Internet age, it is common for individuals to turn to it for information regarding snoring. If you search "apps for snoring" there are more than 11 million "hits." Because many apps are similar, only a few will be discussed here, and by the time you have read this there will be new snoring apps available.

SnoreLab is an example of a readily available app that can be downloaded on any smartphone. An initial trial period is complimentary, then a monthly fee applies if the user chooses to have it for a longer period. SnoreLab records, measures, and tracks snoring. The app is turned on next to the bed when the individual turns in for the night and will display a Snore Score, which tracks when and how loud the snoring was and can be played back for purposes of demonstration (**Fig. 5**). Apps such as SnoreLab allow the individual to document an implemented intervention, such as having an alcoholic beverage before sleep, and evaluate such an effect on their snoring. Although alcohol will most likely make snoring worse, the individual could try sleeping on his or her side to find out whether such an intervention lessens the snoring burden.

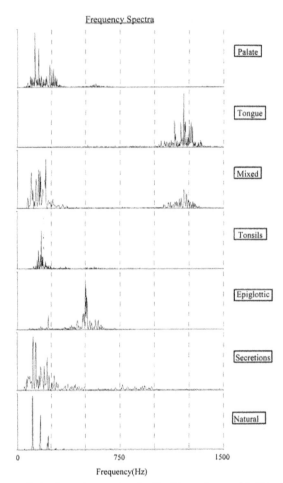

Fig. 4. Frequency analysis of snoring anatomic site. (*From* Agrawal S, Stone P, McGuinness K, et al. Sound frequency analysis and the site of snoring in natural and induced sleep. Clin Otolaryngol Allied Sci. 2002;27(3):162–6; with permission.)

3Snore Control records snoring and either reports the data or activates a "stop snoring" function which, on the iPhone, produces a sound or vibration to quiet the individual.

A new generation of sleep apnea apps is being introduced with the goal of diagnosing OSA from the individual's smartphone or smartwatch. None, at this time, are approved by the Food and Drug Administration (FDA) to diagnose OSA. However, these apps may be helpful in determining whether further testing is warranted.

HEALTH RISKS OF SIMPLE SNORING

There is increasing concern that snoring without the presence of OSA is a health risk and affects the quality of life. Many snorers complain of nonrefreshing sleep and impaired cognitive function.[11] Daytime symptoms may be due to poor sleep efficiency and reduction in sleep time from waking themselves up.

OSA is a known risk factor for atherosclerosis. A study of newly diagnosed OSA patients with no history of cardiovascular disease and snoring were studied with β-mode

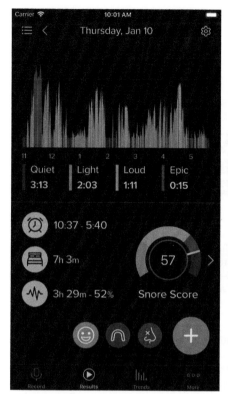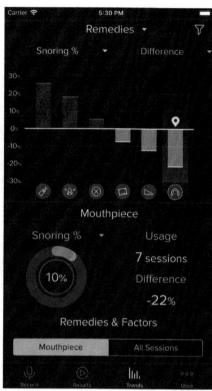

Fig. 5. SnoreLab (snorelab.com) displays graphics that indicate time of snoring, intensity, and tracking over time, the opportunity being that when an individual sleeps on one's back, or has an alcoholic beverage at night, there is feedback regarding the impact on snoring. (*Courtesy of* SnoreLab, London, UK.)

ultrasonography to determine carotid artery intima-media thickness (CCA-IMT).[12] In animal models, the vibratory energy of snoring sounds can be transmitted to the carotid artery, causing endothelial dysfunction and atherosclerosis. After adjusting for age, sex, BMI, metabolic syndrome, and 10-year cardiovascular disease risk score, underlying snoring sounds may cause carotid wall thickening (**Fig. 6**).

In another study, 110 volunteers (snorers and nonsnorers with only mild, nonhypoxic OSA) underwent polysomnography with quantification of snoring, bilateral carotid and femoral artery ultrasonography, and quantification of atherosclerosis and cardiovascular risk factor assessment.[13] Individuals were placed into mild (0%–25% night snoring), moderate (>25%–50% night snoring), or heavy (>50% night snoring) categories of snoring. Heavy snoring was found to increase the risk of carotid atherosclerosis, and this increase was independent of severity of OSA or nocturnal hypoxia.

Another group of patients, who were found to have a snoring problem and no evidence of OSA on polysomnography, were studied by Deeb and colleagues.[14] Fifty-four patients between the ages of 18 and 50 years underwent polysomnography and were found to be nonapneic snorers. They completed the carotid duplex ultrasonography and Snoring Outcomes Survey and were compared according to smoking status, hypertension, diabetes, high cholesterol, and gender. The results

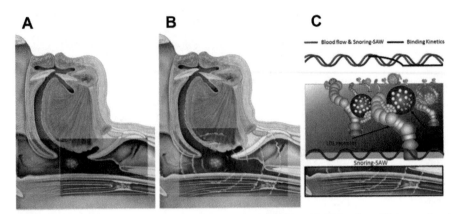

Fig. 6. Possible explanations of snoring and increased CCA-IMT thickening. (*A*) Lower-level obstruction induced local inflammation and oxidative stress. (*B*) Acoustic or vibratory energy of snoring generators causes nearby endothelial damage. (*C*) Surface acoustic wave (SAW) enhances binding kinetics and increases receptor-mediated endocytosis of low-density lipoprotein (LDL). (*From* Lee G-A, Lee L-A, Wang C-Y, et al. The frequency and energy of snoring sounds are associated with common carotid artery intima-media thickness in obstructive sleep apnea patients. Sci Rep. 2016;6:30559.)

demonstrated a statistically significant relation between validated snoring habits and an increased CCA-IMT.

A follow-up study reviewed carotid ultrasonograms at 3 academic vascular laboratories with much larger numbers of patients.[15] A total of 501 patients completed the survey, of whom 243 (49%) had evidence of carotid occlusive disease. On univariate analysis, smoking, hypertension, heart disease, hypercholesterolemia, diabetes, and stroke all correlated with greater than 50% carotid stenosis. Multivariate analysis indicated that snorers were significantly more likely to have carotid disease. Three hundred twenty-seven participants were thought to have primary snoring. On univariate analysis, snorers were found to be significantly more likely to have carotid disease. After adjustment for covariates, snoring was found not to have a significant association with carotid disease. However, multivariate analysis showed snorers to be significantly more likely to have bilateral carotid disease. Snorers were 50% more likely to show carotid stenosis.

BED PARTNER

Snoring is often more of a problem for the bed partner than for the snorer. The bed partner is unable to sleep because of the noise and will nudge the snorer to change position in hopes of alleviating the snoring. Although some snoring is positional, meaning that the snoring lessens with a change in position, it is also possible that by prodding the bed partner to change position the arousal leads to less upper airway muscle relaxation and, subsequently, less snoring. There is also a strong subjective bias in the assessment of snoring by the snorer, bed partner, or observer. A study evaluated objective measurement of snoring, self-perception of snoring by the snorer, and as perceived by the sleep technologist during polysomnography.[16] Based on a snoring rating of none, mild, moderate, or severe, the investigators found that most patients who snored were unaware of their behavior, with a moderate correlation between the technologist's impression and the objective snore index and a poor agreement between the patient's and technologist's subjective impression. This certainly lends credence to the idea that "snoring is in the ear of the beholder."

Ten married couples were studied to determine the effect of snoring on sleep disruption for the partner. Both partners underwent diagnostic polysomnography in the same bed.[17] Midway through the night study, the patient (snorer), all of whom were men, received nasal continuous positive airway pressure (CPAP) adjusted to eliminate snoring. During the CPAP trial, the arousal index of the spouses decreased and their sleep efficiency increased. Over an entire night, this translates to 13% improvement in sleep efficiency and results in an additional 62 minutes of sleep per night for a bed partner of a snorer. The female spouses reported that they habitually slept in the same bed with the snorer, with 8 reporting being awoken nightly by snoring and 7 reporting difficulties returning to sleep because of snoring. It is easy to understand the bed partner's distress: if they are losing an hour of sleep nightly, this translates to an entire night of sleep lost every week and ultimately chronic sleep deprivation.

The intensity of snoring presents the possibility of causing hearing loss in the snorer and the bed partner. As previously mentioned, bed partners of patients with OSA are exposed to environmental noise levels that exceed the limits of nocturnal environmental noise pollution levels recommended by government agencies.[18]

One study evaluated the presence of noise-induced hearing loss for the snorers and their bed partners.[19] Healthy adults between the ages of 35 and 55 years with subjective symptoms of severe snoring were screened to exclude history of noise exposure, ototoxic medications, or previous hearing loss. Audiograms were performed on the snorers and bed partners. The 4 bed partners demonstrated a unilateral hearing loss consistent with noise-induced hearing loss in the ear that was chronically exposed to snoring noise.

WHAT WORSENS SNORING?

It is important, as part of the history taking of snoring, to ask about duration of snoring, weight gain, alcohol consumption, time in bed, and whether the snoring is positional. Having the spouse/bed partner or observer available to answer the questions or help confirm the patient's responses can be invaluable. This is true for many reasons. If there are behavioral factors affecting the snoring, procedural interventions offered may not be successful and the patient will be unhappy. Most procedural interventions are not covered by insurance because snoring is often currently considered a social rather than a medical issue and is treated as if it is "cosmetic." For this reason, many patients will need to pay for the procedures.

LIFESTYLE OR BEHAVIOR

Changes in lifestyle or behavior may be suggested for snorers, and can be very effective.[20] Being overweight or obese contributes to snoring, and a relatively small amount of weight loss can eliminate or alleviate the problem. Although many individuals think of their waist measurement as an indication of being overweight, the neck circumference and even tongue size will decrease when there is weight loss. Many patients will volunteer that when they were 10 lb lighter they didn't snore. Alcohol causes muscle relaxation and, interestingly, it is more pronounced in the tongue than in other areas of the body. The slurred speech that is often noted as an indication of too much alcohol is an example. Advising individuals to eliminate alcohol from their routine may be difficult, but trying it for a week to observe any benefits in their sleep can demonstrate positive outcomes. Given that the use of sedatives to help sleep can cause the same effects as alcohol, diphenhydramine, which is an ingredient of many sleep aids and is often still used for nasal congestion, should be eliminated and replaced with a milder sedating alternative.

TREATMENTS FOR SNORING
Continuous Positive Airway Pressure

CPAP is commonly used for OSA, but for many patients it is the solution to snoring. CPAP is a medical device, and the patient will require a clinical referral to order it through a durable medical equipment supplier or online. Because medical insurance will not cover the costs if there is a negative sleep study for OSA, patients will often be responsible for the cost of the device and supplies. CPAP equipment can be obtained on eBay and via other e-commerce companies.

Oral Appliances

Research shows that an oral appliance can be an effective treatment option for snoring. An oral sleep appliance is worn in the mouth during sleep and fits like a sports mouthguard or an orthodontic retainer. Oral appliances position the jaw in a forward position to help maintain an open upper airway and work similarly to the "jaw thrust" performed by anesthesia when the tongue falls posteriorly and blocks the airway. Titratable oral appliances allow the provider and individual to advance the mandibular portion to achieve maximum benefits. Oral appliances are quiet, portable, and easily cared for, which allows them to be used routinely. However, oral appliances should be fitted by qualified doctors or dentists who are trained and experienced in dental occlusion and associated oral structures. Oral appliances may aggravate temporomandibular joint disease and change dental occlusion; therefore, follow-up is important.[21]

Although many individuals may order oral appliances online because they are less expensive and do not require a visit to a professional, these oral appliances are generally less effective. The over-the-counter or online products are usually a plastic polymer that is placed in boiling water to soften the material. The individual is then instructed to "bite" into the plastic to mold it for fit. Unfortunately, this process does not allow changes to the position of the mandible if the first attempt is insufficient to anteriorly displace the mandible. It is not uncommon to have individuals indicate they have tried oral appliances and that they were ineffective, when in fact the appliance was of poor quality and not custom fitted. More than 100 oral appliances have received FDA clearance.

Any product that keeps the mouth closed enlarges the oropharyngeal airway and decreases resistance and the chances for snoring. Chin Straps and SomniFix (**Fig. 7**) are devices that assist in keeping the mouth closed and are advertised to decrease snoring.

Complementary and Alternative Medicines

Complementary and alternative medicine (CAM) treatments are popular for many conditions, and individuals freely access the Internet as a first step for solutions to issues they are experiencing, often before they consult a medical provider. If one "Googles" snoring, there are 43.7 million results. For obvious reasons only a few of the more common CAM treatments are discussed here, given the many copycat-type devices or preparations available.

Several types of sprays are advertised to improve or eliminate snoring. These sprays are usually "essential oils" that are lightly fragrant volatile substances, which occur in leaves, petals, fruit, and plant roots. "Help Stop Snoring" is such a product, which was

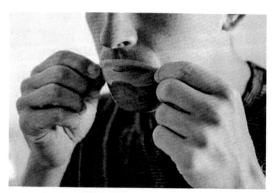

Fig. 7. SomniFix mouth strips (somnifix.com), an over-the-counter remedy, uses an adhesive that seals the lips closed. (*Courtesy of* SomniFix.)

studied in 140 adult snorers.[22] Individuals were randomized to use this spray, gargle, or a placebo. Each snoring volunteer and bed partner completed a "snoring record" that was a 14-day visual analog scale (VAS). This was done for 2 weeks before use to establish baseline snoring threshold. Of the cohort, 82% of patients using the "Help Stop Snoring" spray had partners report a reduction in snoring, 71% using the gargle had a reduction, whereas only 44% of the placebo group reported a decrease in snoring.

Because snoring sound is generated by vibration and resistance in the upper airway, it is feasible that oil-based products increase laminar flow and decrease resistance. In support of this theory, 37 snoring patients and their partners were studied for snoring severity, snoring frequency, AHI, smoking, rhinometry, and BMI.[8] The combination of snoring and high nasal resistance was correlated with habitual snoring. Smoking and mouth breathing are associated with symptoms of dry mouth and throat, which supports the theory that lubrication of the upper airway may improve laminar airflow and decrease resistance.

Nasal Congestion

Individuals with nasal congestion often become mouth breathers, especially at night, when muscle tone decreases and the mouth drops open. When this happens the mandible and tongue swing posteriorly, causing a narrower airway and increased resistance. Snorers seem to have increased nasal resistance in the supine position. The addition of smoking tends to aggravate snoring.[23]

Positional Therapy

Sleeping on one's side often eliminates or lessens snoring and is referred to as positional therapy. During the American War of Independence (1775–1783) and later during World War I, soldiers were advised to wear their rucksacks while sleeping to avoid sleeping on their backs, thus to reduce snoring and avoid detection by the enemy.[24]

Twenty-five adults with positional OSA and snoring were prospectively enrolled in a study to determine whether a head-positioning pillow (HPP) designed for positional therapy could reduce snoring sounds[25] (**Fig. 8**). Subjective snoring severity was measured on a VAS ranging from 0 to 10, and an objective snoring index was used. Both end points were recorded over 3 consecutive nights. Based on BMI, snoring severity and snoring index were significantly lower when the HPP was used. In patients who were overweight, the snoring severity was reduced but the snoring index

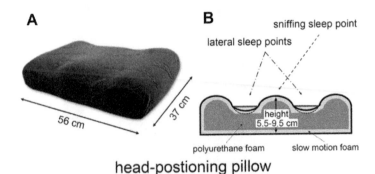

head-postioning pillow

Fig. 8. (*A*) Original image of the HPP pillow. (*B*) Cross-sectional image and materials used for fabricating the HPP pillow. (*From* Chen W-C, Lee L-A, Chen N-H, et al. Treatment of snoring with positional therapy in patients with positional obstructive sleep apnea syndrome. Sci Rep. 2015;5:18188.)

was unchanged. Positional therapy has been shown to be helpful in snorers and should be explored as a treatment approach.

There are several ways to encourage snorers sleep on their side, such as sewing a pocket with a plastic ball in it to the back of a shirt that they wear to bed. When rolling onto their back, they experience an uncomfortable bump that prevents them from staying in that position. There are other commercially devices also available for this purpose, such as elongated pillows or foam wedges that can be placed at the snorers' back when they are on their side so they cannot roll onto their backs. Another approach is using a vibratory device (Night Shift sleep positioner; Advanced Brain Monitoring, Carlsbad, CA), worn around the neck, which incorporates a positional sensor and snoring microphone and delivers a progressively stronger vibrational stimulus to prompt the snorer to shift from the supine position. The device is clinically approved for treatment of OSA and has shown a reduction in the AHI concurrent with a decrease in the arousal index.[26]

Surgical Procedures

There are numerous surgical procedures that have been suggested to improve snoring, none of which, however, have been shown to work for all snorers. Most of the following procedures are presented for treatment of snoring and not for treatment of OSA. Most procedures discussed here are those that can be performed in an outpatient setting with local anesthetic.

In the United States, medical insurance currently does not consider snoring a medical diagnosis that warrants therapy. The following procedures may be considered cosmetic and would not be covered by insurance and, consequently, an out-of-pocket expense for the patient.

Injection snoreplasty

Injection snoreplasty was described by Brietzke and Mair[27] as an office procedure for snoring. Because palatal flutter is the most common cause of snoring, palatal stiffening procedures decrease the vibratory sounds. A well-described sclerotherapy agent, sodium tetradecyl sulfate (Sotradecol), or dehydrated alcohol, is injected into the soft palate to reduce or eliminate palatal flutter snoring. Twenty-five (92%) of 27 patients reported a significant decrease in snoring. There were no significant postinjection complications. A visual analog pain scale confirmed minimal discomfort.

Laser-assisted uvulopalatoplasty

Laser-assisted uvulopalatoplasty (LAUP) was introduced in the 1980s as an alternative to uvulopalatopharyngoplasty that could be performed in the office with the patient under local anesthesia.[28] It has fallen out of favor because it is more painful than other more recently developed procedures, and may require several procedures with expensive laser equipment. The soft palate and uvula are injected with local anesthetic and the laser is used to shorten the uvula and soft palate. Care is taken to not experience collateral thermal injury to the posterior pharyngeal wall that would possibly result in circumferential fibrosis and nasopharyngeal stenosis.

Cautery-assisted palatal stiffening operation

The cautery-assisted palatal stiffening operation (CAPSO) for snorers was described by Mair and Day.[29] CAPSO is a mucosal palatal surgery that induces a midline palatal scar which stiffens the floppy palate. A cohort of 206 consecutive patients underwent CAPSO over an 18-month period, followed by office examination and telephone evaluation. The success rate was initially 92%, which decreased to 77% after 1 year.

Palatal radiofrequency ablation

Palatal radiofrequency ablation for the treatment of snoring was described by Powell and colleagues.[30] The study evaluates the effects of radiofrequency energy (RFe) to the palate of patients with sleep-disordered breathing with a respiratory disturbance index of less than 15, or what would be considered snoring without OSA. Volunteers enrolled in this investigation were 18 to 65 years of age and were seeking treatment for symptomatic chronic (habitual) snoring and reported symptoms of daytime sleepiness. Subjective snoring scores decreased by a mean of 77% accompanied by improved mean Epworth sleepiness scores. A systematic literature review of radiofrequency ablation of the palate by Bäck and colleagues[31] included 30 articles that met the criteria. The risk of adverse events and the risk of side effects were small and there was a reduction in snoring in the short term.

SUMMARY

The "when and why" of the treatment of snoring is decided when the individual comes to the physician seeking relief. It is important to evaluate any individuals who seek treatment for snoring with a sleep study, if possible, to eliminate the diagnosis of OSA. There is no one treatment that eliminates snoring in all patients. Obtaining a history and physical examination can assist in determining which therapies may be helpful as a first step, but multiple different interventions may be necessary to achieve success. As in many medical conditions, the idea of "step therapy" and incremental improvement should be considered as a pathway to success and peaceful coexistence for bed partners.

More research is being carried out to determine the long-term effects on health of snoring, which it is hoped will transition it from a "social nuisance" to a medical condition that deserves treatment. The bed partners of snorers will also ultimately benefit when all concerned are able to enjoy a "silent night."

DISCLOSURE

The author has nothing to disclose.

REFERENCES

1. Definition of SNORE. Merriam-webster.com. 2019. Available at: https://www.merriam-webster.com/dictionary/snore. Accessed October 1, 2019.
2. History of the OED | Oxford English Dictionary. Oxford English Dictionary. 2019. Available at: https://public.oed.com/history/. Accessed October 1, 2019.
3. Why does Z stand for snoring?. Washington City Paper. 2019. Available at: https://www.washingtoncitypaper.com/columns/straight-dope/article/13042858/why-does-z-stand-for-snoring-and-how-do-other. Accessed October 1, 2019.
4. Gavriely N, Jensen O. Theory and measurement of snores. J Appl Physiol 1993;74:2828–37.
5. Lee LA, Yu JF, Lo YL, et al. Energy types of snoring sounds in patients with obstructive sleep apnea syndrome: a preliminary observation. PLoS One 2012;7(12):e53481.
6. Maimon N, Hanly PJ. Does snoring intensity correlate with the severity of obstructive sleep apnea? J Clin Sleep Med 2010;6(5):475–8.
7. Fiz JA, Abad J, Jané R, et al. Acoustic analysis of snoring sound in patients with simple snoring and obstructive sleep apnoea. Eur Respir J 1996;9(11):2365–70.
8. Wilson K, Mulrooney T, Gawtry RR. Snoring: an acoustic monitoring technique. Laryngoscope 1985;95(10):1174–7.
9. Agrawal S, Stone P, McGuinness K, et al. Sound frequency analysis and the site of snoring in natural and induced sleep. Clin Otolaryngol Allied Sci 2002;27(3):162–6.
10. Herzog M, Schmidt A, Bremert T, et al. Analysed snoring sounds correlate to obstructive sleep disordered breathing. Eur Arch Otorhinolaryngol 2008;265(1):105–13.
11. Hoffstein V, Mateika JH, Mateika S. Snoring and sleep architecture. Am Rev Respir Dis 1991;143(1):92–6.
12. Lee GS, Lee LA, Wang CY, et al. The frequency and energy of snoring sounds are associated with common carotid artery intima-media thickness in obstructive sleep apnea patients. Sci Rep 2016;6:30559.
13. Lee SA, Amis TC, Byth K, et al. Heavy snoring as a cause of carotid artery atherosclerosis. Sleep 2008;31(9):1207–13.
14. Deeb R, Judge P, Peterson E, et al. Snoring and carotid artery intima-media thickness. Laryngoscope 2014;124(6):1486–91.
15. Deeb R, Smeds MR, Bath J, et al. Snoring and carotid artery disease: A new risk factor emerges. Laryngoscope 2019;129(1):265–8.
16. Hoffstein V, Mateika S, Anderson D. Snoring: is it in the ear of the beholder? Sleep 1994;17(6):522–6.
17. Beninati W, Harris CD, Herold DL, et al. The effect of snoring and obstructive sleep apnea on the sleep quality of bed partners. Mayo Clin Proc 1999;74(10):955–8.
18. Hammer MS, Swinburn TK, Neitzel RL. Environmental noise pollution in the United States: developing an effective public health response. Environ Health Perspect 2014;122(2):115–9.
19. Sardesai MG, Tan AK, Fitzpatrick M. Noise-induced hearing loss in snores and their bed partners. J Otolaryngol 2003;32(3):141–5.
20. Counter P, Wilson JA. The management of simple snoring. Sleep Med Rev 2004;8(6):433–41.

21. Ramar K, Dort LC, Katz SG, et al. Clinical practice guideline for the treatment of obstructive sleep apnea and snoring with oral appliance therapy: an update for 2015. J Clin Sleep Med 2015;11(7):773–82.
22. Prichard AJ. The use of essential oils to treat snoring. Phytother Res 2004;18(9): 696–9.
23. Virkkula P, Bachour A, Hytönen M, et al. Patient- and bed partner-reported symptoms, smoking, and nasal resistance in sleep-disordered breathing. Chest 2005; 128(4):2176–82.
24. Ravesloot MJ, van Maanen JP, Dun L, et al. The undervalued potential of positional therapy in position-dependent snoring and obstructive sleep apnea—a review of the literature. Sleep Breath 2013;17(1):39–49.
25. Chen WC, Lee LA, Chen NH, et al. Treatment of snoring with positional therapy in patients with positional obstructive sleep apnea syndrome. Sci Rep 2015;5: 18188.
26. Levendowski DJ, Seagraves S, Popovic D, et al. Assessment of a neck-based treatment and monitoring device for positional obstructive sleep apnea. J Clin Sleep Med 2014;10(8):863–71.
27. Brietzke SE, Mair EA. Injection snoreplasty: how to treat snoring without all the pain and expense. Otolaryngol Head Neck Surg 2001;124(5):503–10.
28. Kamami YV. Laser CO_2 for snoring. Preliminary results. Acta Otorhinolaryngol Belg 1990;44(4):451–6.
29. Mair EA, Day RH. Cautery-assisted palatal stiffening operation. Otolaryngol Head Neck Surg 2000;122(4):547–56.
30. Powell NB, Riley RW, Troell RJ, et al. Radiofrequency volumetric tissue reduction of the palate in subjects with sleep-disordered breathing. Chest 1998;113(5): 1163–74.
31. Bäck LJ, Hytönen ML, Roine RP, et al. Radiofrequency ablation treatment of soft palate for patients with snoring: a systematic review of effectiveness and adverse effects. Laryngoscope 2009;119(6):1241–50.

Sleep Studies Interpretation and Application

Robert Hiensch, MD*, David M. Rapoport, MD

KEYWORDS

- Polysomnography • Home sleep apnea test • Obstructive sleep apnea

KEY POINTS

- Patients with snoring, nocturnal gasping or choking, and unexplained excessive daytime sleepiness should be evaluated for obstructive sleep apnea. Obesity, retrognathia, and increased nasal resistance are risk factors for obstructive sleep apnea.
- Obstructive sleep apnea is associated with certain cardiovascular conditions, such as atrial fibrillation and hypertension.
- Polysomnography is the gold standard for diagnosing obstructive sleep apnea.
- Home sleep apnea testing is an alternative, less-costly method of diagnosing obstructive sleep apnea in nonmedically complex patients who are at high risk for the disease.
- The results of the sleep study help define the role of upper airway surgery to treat obstructive sleep apnea.

INTRODUCTION

The development of polysomnography (PSG) in the 1960s helped create the new medical specialty of sleep medicine. The subsequent discovery that obstructive sleep apnea (OSA) was both common and medically serious, yet effectively treatable with continuous positive airway pressure (CPAP), fueled its explosive growth. PSG remains the gold standard for the evaluation of not just sleep-related breathing disorders, but most clinical sleep disorders. The technology behind sleep studies continues to evolve and influence the approach to the growing population of patients with sleep complaints. This review describes the indications for sleep studies and their application in the evaluation of OSA from the point of view of the otorhinolaryngologist.

INDICATIONS FOR TESTING

OSA is a common condition. Depending on the definition of disease and method of testing, prevalence rates range from 2% to 9% in women and 4% to 24% in

Department of Medicine, Division of Pulmonary, Critical Care, and Sleep Medicine, Icahn School of Medicine at Mount Sinai, 1 Gustave L. Levy Place, Box 1232, New York, NY 10029, USA
* Corresponding author.
E-mail address: robert.hiensch@gmail.com

Otolaryngol Clin N Am 53 (2020) 367–383
https://doi.org/10.1016/j.otc.2020.02.012
0030-6665/20/© 2020 Elsevier Inc. All rights reserved.
oto.theclinics.com

men.[1,2] Subgroups, such as the bariatric population, have an even higher prevalence rate.[3] Furthermore, although OSA rates are increasing in concert with rising rates of obesity, a large proportion of those affected are undiagnosed.[3,4] Despite the high prevalence, the United States Preventive Services Task Force does not recommend screening for OSA in asymptomatic adults, although clinical case-finding may be worthwhile.[5-7] Therefore, it is important to understand the risk factors, signs, symptoms, and comorbidities relevant to OSA.

Most risk factors for OSA predispose to disease by reducing the size of the pharynx or increasing airway collapsibility.[3] Obesity is the most important risk factor.[8] In the morbidly obese (body mass index $\geq$40 kg/m^2), prevalence rates as high as 88% have been reported.[9] OSA is less common in women, although the gender gap narrows after menopause. It also increases with advancing age in a manner independent of weight gain.[3] Craniofacial or upper airway abnormalities, such as micrognathia, adenotonsillar hypertrophy, and nasal congestion, also increase the risk of OSA.

Assessment of symptomatology is of utmost importance in the evaluation of OSA since symptoms help guide both the evaluation and treatment of the disease. Unfortunately, many of the symptoms of OSA are nonspecific. OSA should be considered in any person presenting with unexplained sleepiness, particularly if there are additional risk factors. Sleepiness not due to OSA is common in the general population, however, and it may be easily confused with fatigue. Accompanying complaints, such as snoring, nocturia, unrefreshing sleep, morning headaches, and poor concentration and memory may narrow the differential to OSA.[3,10] Nocturnal choking or gasping is the most useful individual symptom, with a specificity of 84%, although the sensitivity is only 52%.[11] Some patients may not report nocturnal symptoms, such as snoring, if there is no bed partner. Even diurnal symptoms, such as sleepiness may not be perceived by the patient if it has been long standing and the patient has adjusted his or her lifestyle around it. Women with OSA often manifest with insomnia and mood changes, which may be a reason for underdiagnosis in this population.[12]

The physical examination in a patient with suspected OSA focuses on recognizing risk factors for or identifying a narrow or collapsible airway. As mentioned, obesity is the most important objective finding, and the prevalence of OSA increases as markers of obesity, such as body mass index, neck circumference, and waist-to-hip ratio, increase.[13] Increased nasopharyngeal resistance due to septal deviation or turbinate hypertrophy also increases the risk of OSA due to the Starling resistor model. Higher Mallampati scores correlate with the presence and severity of OSA. Dental overjet, macroglossia, mandibular insufficiency, and a vaulted hard palate are other physical examination findings that increase the risk of OSA.[13-15] Flexible fiberoptic laryngoscopy visualizes the whole upper aerodigestive tract and may identify sites of potential obstruction and surgical intervention in patients with OSA. Findings, such as mega-epiglottis and modified Cormack-Lehane score of 2 or more are independent predictors of moderate to severe OSA.[16] Cephalometrics can also identify potential sources of obstruction but noninvasively. Such assessment methods occur during wake, however. Despite their utility to suggest OSA during the daytime evaluation, to date no test performed awake has shown acceptable sensitivity to rule out OSA, and the specificity of most tests remains suboptimal. Obstructive physiology during drug-induced sleep endoscopy (DISE) correlates with obstructive events that occur during natural sleep; however, DISE is more invasive and the utility of DISE to predict surgical outcomes is less clear.[17-19]

Many comorbid diseases are associated with OSA. These include hypertension, stroke, atrial fibrillation, congestive heart failure, coronary artery disease, renal disease, and chronic obstructive pulmonary disease. OSA is also more common in acromegaly, polycystic ovarian disease, and certain genetic disorders, such as Down syndrome and Pierre Robin syndrome. Certainly, anyone presenting with symptoms of OSA and any of these conditions should be tested for OSA.[13] Whether asymptomatic individuals with these conditions should be evaluated for OSA is debated.[6,20–23]

A variety of clinical tools, questionnaires, and prediction algorithms aim to predict the presence of OSA in adults (**Table 1**). Although such tools may aid in identifying patients at higher or lower risk of OSA, they are of insufficient diagnostic accuracy by themselves to replace objective testing with sleep studies in most patients. The most important limitation is low specificity. Misdiagnoses can lead to harm by delaying or depriving patients with OSA of therapy and lead to initiation of unnecessary therapy in those without OSA.[7]

Testing for OSA should occur after a comprehensive sleep evaluation and must be adequately followed up. This ensures that the appropriate study is administered and therapy is delivered properly. In situations that require expedited evaluation of OSA, a clinical pathway that includes a focused evaluation of sleep apnea, questionnaires that capture clinically relevant data, and follow-up with a sleep physician may be acceptable.[7]

POLYSOMNOGRAPHY

Laboratory-based attended PSG is the comprehensive monitoring and evaluation of multiple physiologic parameters, including sleep, during a period of sleep. It is considered the gold standard to diagnose OSA and evaluate its severity, not to mention most other sleep disorders. In addition to audio and visual monitoring, PSG records a variety of physiologic parameters during the sleep period (**Table 2**).

A brief overview of the technical components of PSG is necessary to appreciate the indications for and interpretations of sleep studies. To detect and stage sleep, PSG uses 1 to 3 electroencephalogram (EEG) derivations over the frontal, central, and occipital head regions, electrooculography (EOG) and submental electromyography (EMG) to

Table 1
Clinical tools used for the diagnosis of obstructive sleep apnea

Clinical Tool	Composition	Populations Studied	Sensitivity (AHI ≥5) (%)	Specificity (AHI ≥5) (%)
Berlin Questionnaire	11 questions divided into 3 categories	Middle-aged, overweight/ obese, mostly men	76	45
Epworth Sleepiness Scale	8 self-reported questions assessing propensity for daytime sleepiness or dozing	Middle-aged, overweight/ obese, mostly men	27–72	50–76
STOP-BANG	4 yes/no questions and 4 clinical attributes	Middle-aged, obese men	93	36

Data from Kapur VK, Auckley DH, Chowdhuri S, et al. Clinical practice guideline for diagnostic testing for adult obstructive sleep apnea: an American Academy of Sleep Medicine Clinical Practice Guideline. J Clin Sleep Med. 2017;13(3):479-504.

Table 2
Physiologic parameters studied in standard nocturnal polysomnography

Parameter	Sensors	Purpose
Electroencephalography	Frontal, central, occipital leads with mastoid process reference lead	Stage sleep, detect epileptiform activity
Electrooculography	Outer canthi leads with mastoid process reference lead	Stage sleep (specifically stage R)
Electromyography	Submental surface electrodes Anterior tibial surface electrodes	Stage sleep (specifically stage R), detect REM without atonia, detect periodic limb movements and other movement abnormalities
Airflow	Nasal cannula pressure transducer Oronasal thermal sensor PAP device (titration study)	Detection of hypopneas and RERAs Detection of apneas Detection of apneas, hypopneas, and RERAs
PAP device pressure, leak, tidal volume (titration study)	PAP device flow and pressure sensors	Detect pressure, leak, tidal volume
Snoring	Microphone, piezoelectric sensor	Detect snoring
Respiratory effort	Chest and abdomen respiratory inductance plethysmography belts	Classify respiratory events as obstructive, central, or mixed
Arterial oxygen saturation	Pulse oximetry	Detect hypoxemia
Ventilation	End-tidal Pco_2 or transcutaneous Pco_2 monitoring	Detect hypoventilation
Electrocardiogram	Modified lead II	Monitor cardiac rate and rhythm
Position	Accelerometer, video monitors	Detect position
Behavior	Audio, video monitors	Detect parasomnias, abnormal behaviors, seizures

Adapted from Meliana V, Chung F, Li CK, Singh M. Interpretation of sleep studies for patients with sleep-disordered breathing: What the anesthesiologist needs to know. Can J Anesth. 2018;65(1):62; with permission.

stage sleep/wake and divide sleep into stages, including light (nonrapid eye movement [NREM] stages 1–2), deep (NREM stage 3), and rapid eye movement (REM) sleep. Respiratory monitoring typically includes surrogate measures of airflow using nasal pressure transducers and oronasal thermocouples, respiratory effort using chest and abdominal effort belts, pulse oximetry, and a snoring microphone. End-tidal or transcutaneous CO_2 monitoring may be included. A modified lead II electrocardiogram detects heart rate and rhythm. Body position may be determined using a position sensor and verified using visual recording. Audiovisual recording further aids in the diagnosis of parasomnias. In PSG where CPAP is being used, PAP device pressure, leak, and flow can be measured in place of thermocouples or nasal pressure transducers.[10]

The parameters are digitally recorded under the observation of a sleep technologist who monitors the quality of the signals and intervenes on issues as they arise. After study completion, the collected data are aggregated and scored.[24] Scoring begins with analyzing each 30-s window (called an epoch) of EEG, EOG, and EMG signals and categorizing it as wake or sleep, and, if sleep, what stage of sleep. Sleep and wake are staged according to the American Academy for Sleep Medicine (AASM) Manual for the Scoring of Sleep and Associated Events (hereinafter referred to as the AASM Manual), which serves as the definitive reference for scoring PSG.[25] Depending on the characteristics of the EEG, EOG, and EMG signals, sleep is subcategorized into NREM and REM sleep. NREM sleep is further divided into stage N1, N2, and N3 sleep. Stage N1 represents a transitional state between wake and sleep. Frequent arousals from sleep, due to OSA, for example, will result in high amounts of stage N1. Most sleep for normal adults consists of stage N2. Stage N3 represents the deepest stage of sleep and is most restorative. It is reduced in cases of OSA. REM sleep, or stage R, is characterized by an EEG pattern resembling wake but with skeletal muscle hypotonia on EMG and rapid eye movements on EOG. The cardiopulmonary system is most unstable during stage R with cardiac arrhythmias, irregular breathing, and respiratory events being more common and more severe. Arousals are defined as brief increases in EEG frequency (and increase in EMG tone for stage R) to that resembling wake EEG. They are a normal part of sleep but become pathologically increased due to OSA and other causes of sleep fragmentation. A high arousal index is usually associated with higher stage N1 and less consolidated (ie, continuous) sleep, which is often associated with symptoms of daytime sleepiness and decreased psychomotor performance.[25]

The scoring of respiratory events is also performed according to the AASM Manual. Rules differ for adults and children. Respiratory events are classified into apneas, hypopneas, and respiratory effort-related arousals (RERAs). For adults, apneas are defined as a ≥90% drop in signal excursion from pre-event baseline on the oronasal thermal sensor or PAP flow tracing for 10 seconds or more. There need not be an accompanying physiologic response (ie, a change in oxygen saturation or EEG arousal), although they are often present. Apneas can be subclassified as obstructive when inspiratory efforts can be detected, most often from persistent thoracoabdominal respiratory inductance plethysmography belt signal excursion during the event. An apnea is classified as central when effort is absent throughout the period of absent airflow. Mixed apneas demonstrate respiratory effort only in the latter portion of the event after an initial portion of absent inspiratory effort (**Fig. 1**),[25] but are generally treated as a variant of obstructive apneas. Hypopneas are reductions in airflow that do not meet apnea criteria but result in a measurable physiologic consequence. The definition of how and what defines "reduction" and "physiologic consequences" has evolved over time with changes in sensor technology and a better appreciation of the pathophysiology of sleep-disordered breathing. This "floating metric," however, has led to considerable confusion in clinical practice and in the literature, particularly when comparing studies that used different definitions.[26] The current recommended definition for hypopnea according the AASM Manual is a ≥30% reduction in peak signal excursion as detected by the nasal pressure transducer or PAP device flow for ≥10 seconds. This must be accompanied by an arousal and/or a ≥3% oxygen desaturation. An alternate "acceptable" definition specifies that the accompanying physiologic change is a ≥4% oxygen desaturation.[25] Hypopneas are often not scored as obstructive or central because respiratory effort, if defined according to the simple presence or absence of thoracoabdominal signal excursion, is present in both circumstances. An esophageal balloon distinguishes between central and obstructive

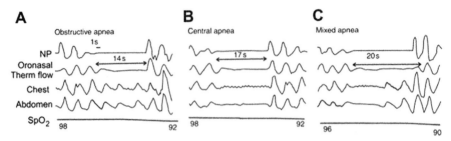

Fig. 1. Obstructive, central, and mixed apneas. Oronasal thermal sensor demonstrates absent or minimal airflow. In obstructive apnea (A), effort is persistent throughout as demonstrated by movement in the chest and abdominal belts. In central apnea (B), there is minimal excursion in the chest and abdominal belts, suggesting that there is no effort to initiate breaths. In mixed apnea (C), an initial portion of absent effort to breathe is followed by effort as manifested by excursion in the chest and abdominal belts only in the second half of the apnea. (From Berry RB, Wagner MH. Respiratory event definitions in adults. In: Sleep medicine pearls. 3rd edition. Philadelphia: Elsevier Saunders; 2015. p. 125; with permission.)

hypopneas by measuring transpulmonary pressure, which reflects effort. However, esophageal balloons are not routinely placed in clinical PSG. Clues that suggest that hypopneas are obstructive include the presence of snoring, prolongation of inspiratory time, flattening of the inspiratory arm of the nasal pressure or PAP device flow (called inspiratory flow limitation), and thoracoabdominal paradox. Inspiratory flow limitation correlates well with increased effort as measured by the esophageal balloon although the tracing does not quantify the degree of respiratory effort (**Fig. 2**).[27] A RERA is a sequence of breaths lasting $\geq$10 seconds that do not meet the criteria for apnea or hypopnea but have increased respiratory effort and lead to an arousal from sleep.[25] With the change by the AASM Manual to include arousals as part of the recommended hypopnea definition, many sleep laboratories reporting the recommended version of the apnea-hypopnea index (AHI) no longer score RERAs.

Other less-frequent breathing phenomena may also occur. Hypoventilation, defined as a sustained reduction in breathing resulting in an increase of arterial Pco_2, may be observed in the morbidly obese, patients with neuromuscular disease, or the pediatric population, among others. Sustained hypoxemia that arises or worsens during sleep in the absence of discrete respiratory events is often assumed to be caused by hypoventilation. Sustained inspiratory flow limitation, although not defined in the AASM Manual, is commonly seen in pregnancy and pediatrics. It manifests as long periods of inspiratory flow limited breathing without intervening scorable respiratory events. Efforts at standardizing the definition of inspiratory flow limitation by consensus have recently been published by the American Thoracic Society.[28] Cheyne-Stokes breathing is a type of central sleep apnea that is usually seen in patients with congestive heart failure, atrial fibrillation, or stroke. See **Box 1** for the definitions of respiratory events.

A variety of other findings that are not related to respiratory phenomena are scored by sleep technologists. These include limb movements, muscle tone, behavioral abnormalities, and cardiac dysrhythmias. Some of these can lead to clinical sequelae that overlap with those due to OSA.

THE SLEEP REPORT

After scoring is complete, a sleep physician reviews the study and, integrating information from the clinical history, interprets and provides recommendations in a sleep

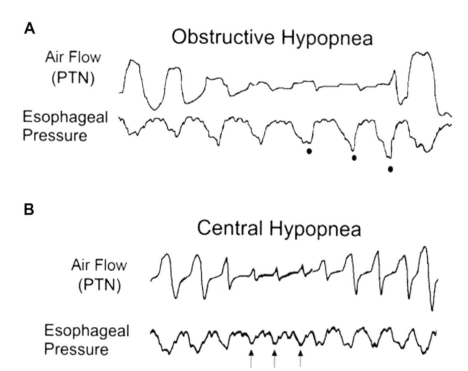

Fig. 2. Hypopneas are ≥30% reductions in airflow on the nasal cannula pressure transducer that do not meet apnea criteria. The presence of inspiratory flattening, thoracoabdominal paradox, and snoring in an obstructive hypopnea (*A*) suggests an obstructive cause, which is confirmed by the increasing negative values noted on the esophageal manometer (*dots*). In central hypopnea (*B*), these features are absent and esophageal pressure remains constant (*arrows*). (*From* Berry RB, Wagner MH. Respiratory event definitions in adults. In: Sleep medicine pearls. 3rd edition. Philadelphia: Elsevier Saunders; 2015. p. 127; with permission.)

study report. This contains the results of the respiratory and nonrespiratory parameters and a summary statement by the sleep physician related to the clinical history and any sleep diagnoses that are identified. It is divided into several parts.

Background

A report starts with demographic data and a brief history that describes the clinical context of the sleep study. It is important to note the type of study performed, which parameters were used, and the presence of any treatment intervention. PSGs can be broadly classified as diagnostic, interventional, or split-night studies. A diagnostic study serves to diagnose disease. An interventional study is performed to observe the effect of and/or optimize an active intervention, such as PAP, oral appliance therapy, or hypoglossal nerve stimulation. A split-night study is usually reserved for cases of severe OSA that are clearly evident in the first few hours of diagnostic testing, which is then followed by implementation of therapy, most often PAP.

Sleep

A summary of the salient features of sleep quality, quantity, and macro-architecture identifies whether sleep was frequently disrupted by respiratory events or otherwise.

Box 1
Definition of respiratory events according to the AASM Manual for the Scoring of Sleep and Associated Events

Apnea	$\geq$90% reduction in oronasal thermal sensor for $\geq$10 s
	Obstructive: continued inspiratory effort throughout the apnea
	Central: absent inspiratory effort throughout the apnea
	Mixed: absent inspiratory effort initially, followed by resumption of effort
Hypopnea	$\geq$30% reduction in nasal cannula pressure transducer for $\geq$10 s associated with either:
	(Recommended) a $\geq$3% oxygen desaturation and/or arousal, OR
	(Acceptable and widely used) a $\geq$4% oxygen desaturation
Respiratory Effort-Related Arousal	Sequence of breaths not meeting other definition of hypopnea, but lasting $\geq$10 s and leading to an arousal with:
	Increased respiratory effort, OR
	Flattening of inspiratory portion of the nasal pressure
Hypoventilation	Increase in P_{CO_2} to a value of >55 mm Hg for $\geq$10 min, OR
	$\geq$10 mm Hg increase in P_{CO_2} during sleep to >50 mm Hg for $\geq$10 min
Cheyne-Stokes breathing	$\geq$3 episodes of consecutive central apneas and/or central hypopneas separated by a crescendo and decrescendo change in breathing amplitude with a cycle length $\geq$40 s, AND
	$\geq$5 central apneas and/or central hypopneas per hour of sleep with the crescendo/decrescendo breathing pattern over $\geq$2 h of monitoring

Data from Berry RB, Brooks R, Gamaldo CE, et al. The AASM Manual for the Scoring of Sleep and Associated Events: Rules, Terminology and Technical Specifications. Version 2.4. Darien, Illinois: American Academy of Sleep Medicine; 2017.

A high amount of stage N1, frequent stage shifts, a high arousal index, and decreased stage R or stage N3 are all frequently seen in OSA.[29] Although the sleep center environment may disturb sleep in some, generally accepted normative values are provided in **Table 3**. Fragmented sleep and arousal indices correlate with subjective and objective measures of sleepiness.[30,31] Adults should enter sleep through NREM and then cycle between NREM and REM sleep approximately every 90 to 100 minutes. A typical healthy young adult will have 4 to 5 of these sleep cycles. Early in the sleep period, NREM stage 2 is often followed by stage N3, which decreases in amount during subsequent cycles as the night progresses. REM stage, on the other hand, increases in quantity and comes to dominate the NREM-REM cycle in the early morning hours. Sleep architecture is subject to many influences, including medications, comorbid disease, and the testing state itself. Certain findings, such as a sleep onset REM period, are highly unusual and should be pointed out by the interpreting sleep physician.[32]

Respiratory

A narrative describing the apneas, hypopneas, and RERAs observed during the study is often the portion of the study of greatest interest to otorhinolaryngologists. The hallmark of OSA (also called obstructive sleep apnea hypopnea syndrome) is the repetitive complete or partial collapse of the upper airway during sleep, which is what occurs during an apnea, hypopnea, and RERA (**Box 2**).[33] This is quantified by the AHI, which divides the sum of apneas, hypopneas, and RERAs by the hours of sleep. Older studies may report the respiratory disturbance index (RDI) and this was previously synonymous with AHI or was occasionally used to include RERAs. Because RERAs are now incorporated into the AHI, this definition should not be used for the RDI. The preceding discussion highlights the importance of knowing which definition of

Table 3
Means with 95% CIs for total sleep time, sleep efficiency, wake after sleep onset, and duration of sleep stages for total simple and by age, sex, and night of sleep study based on random effects models

	Total Sleep Time, min	Sleep Efficiency	Wake After Sleep Onset, min	Duration of Sleep Stages (Percentage of Total Sleep Time)			
				N1	N2	N3	REM
Total sample	394.6 (388 4–400.8); k-158	85.7% (84 8–86.6); k-147	48.2 (43.8–52.6); k-94	7%–9% (7.3–8 5); k-104	51.4% (50.2–52.6); k-104	20.4% (19 0–21 8); k-107	19.0% (18 5–19 6); k-108
Mean age, years							
18–34	410.6 (404 5–416.6); k-76	89.0% (88.0–90.0); k-65	32.1 (28.2–36.1); k-42	6.0% (5.3–6.7); k-38;	51.3% (49.6–52.9); k-39	21.4% (20.0–22.8); k-42	19.8% (18.8–20.8); k-44
35–49	386.6 (371.4–401.9); k-32	85.4% (83.7–87.1); k-35	51.1 (41.1–61.1); k-22	8.0% (6.9–9.2); k-23	52.2% (50 6–53 8); k-24	20.4% (18.5–22.2); k-23	19.3% (18.2–20.3); k-24
50–64	372.0 (358.1–85.89); k-26	83.2% (81.0–85.4); k-27	64.0 (55.1–72.9); k-17	8.7% (7.3–10.0); k-22	52.8% (49.8–55.8); k-22	18.1% (15.0–21.2); k-23	18.7% (17.8–19.6); k-23
65–79	346.0 (326.7–365.4); k-17	77.5% (73.0–81.9); k-16	77.1 (57.3–96.9); k-12	9.3% (7.0–11.6); k-11;	53.3% (50.0–56.7); k-11	19.9% (17.8–22.1); k-11	17.7% (l6.9-18.5); k-10
≥80	198.6 (142.5–254.7); k-1	45.7% (33.7–57.7); k-1	NA	27.5% (15.0–40.0); k-1	43.5% (37.8–49.2); k-1	19.1% (8.3–29.9); k-l	9.9% (4.4–15.4); k-l
Sex							
Both	405.2 (398.8–411.7); k-l01	86.7% (85.5–87.8); k-96	43.3 (37.9–48.8); k-56	9.7% (8.7–10.6); k-59	50.6% (48.7–52.5); k-59	19.5% (17.5–21.4); k-62	19.2% (18.5–19.9); k-63
Men only	374.6 (357.3–392.0); k-30	84.3% (82.0–86.6); k-27	51.8 (42.1–61.4); k-20	5.3% (4.5–6.1); k-23	52.1% (50.2–53.9); k-24	21.0% (19.5–22.4); k-24	19.9% (18.5–21.2); k-24
Women only	356.0 (337.3–374.8); k-l 9	84.1% (81.6–86.5); k-19	55.0 (46.3–63.7); k-17	4.2% (3.6–4.7); k-16	55.1% (54.0–56.3); k-16	22.1% (20.8–23.4); k-17	18.6% (17.9–19.3); k-17

(continued on next page)

376   Hiensch & Rapoport

Table 3
(continued)

	Total Sleep Time, min	Sleep Efficiency	Wake After Sleep Onset, min	Duration of Sleep Stages (Percentage of Total Sleep Time)			
				N1	N2	N3	REM
Night of sleep study							
First night	371.6 (361.8–381.3); k-89	84.2% (83.0–85.4); k-88	52.7 (46.7–58.7); k-57	7.0% (6.4–7.5); k-63	52.1% (50.8–53.3); k-69	20.7% (19.6–21.8); k-69	18.3% (17.7–18.8); k-68
Second night or later	419.7 (412.0–427.4); k-48	89.3% (88.0–90.5); k-39	37.9 (30.6–45.2); k-26	6.9% (5.6–8.3); k-23	48.2% (45.7–50.8); k-24	22.3% (18.5–26.2); k-25	21.4% (20.0–22.7); k-26

Variable k represents the number of control groups combined to reach the pooled estimate, the corresponding number of participants for each estimate is included in the appendix. Some studies included more than one control group.

Abbreviations: NA, no studies available at this age cut off; REM, rapid eye movement.

Reprinted with permission from Elsevier (Boulos MI, Jairam T, Kendzerska T, et al. Normal polysomnography parameters in healthy adults: a systematic review and meta-analysis. Lancet Respir Med. 2019;7(6):537).

Box 2
The definition of obstructive sleep apnea per the International Classification of Sleep Disorders, Third Edition requires either A or B to be satisfied

A.
$\geq$1 of:
1. Sleepiness, nonrestorative sleep, fatigue, or insomnia symptoms
2. Breath holding, gasping, or choking
3. Habitual snoring, breathing interruptions, or both during sleep
4. Hypertension, mood disorder, cognitive dysfunction, coronary artery disease, stroke, congestive heart failure, atrial fibrillation, or type 2 diabetes mellitus

AND
1. AHI $\geq$5 (predominantly obstructive respiratory events [obstructive apneas, mixed apneas, hypopneas, or RERAs] per hour of sleep during a polysomnography or home sleep apnea test)

B.
1. AHI $\geq$15 (predominantly obstructive respiratory events [obstructive apneas, mixed apneas, hypopneas, or RERAs] per hour of sleep during a polysomnography or home sleep apnea test)

Adapted from American Academy of Sleep Medicine. International Classification of Sleep Disorders. 3rd ed. Darien,IL: American Academy of Sleep Medicine; 2014. p. 63; with permission.

---

hypopnea was used for scoring a given sleep study, and this should always be explicitly stated. Depending on the definition used to define a hypopnea (4% or 3% and/or arousal), the AHI may vary considerably in a given individual and could classify the same individual as being normal or having disease.[34–36] Reporting an AHI without saying the measure of hypopnea is akin to saying the speed limit is 60 but not specifying whether it is in kilometers per hour or miles per hour. This is especially important when comparing test results from different time periods or from different sleep laboratories.

The AHI is an important measure of OSA and severity because it has been found to correlate, albeit modestly, with morbidity and mortality, and lowering the AHI through therapy results in improvements in symptoms and certain cardiovascular outcomes.[37,38] Based on consensus, severity of OSA is defined according to the cutoffs listed in **Table 4**.[13] Although PAP is considered first-line therapy for all severities of OSA, surgical intervention is an alternative option for mild OSA, and can be considered for moderate to severe OSA if PAP is not tolerated.[13] Besides symptoms, the AHI is the most reported outcome measure in studies of surgical interventions. A typical surgical "cure" is a decrease in the AHI by $\geq$50% to a level of $\leq$20 events/h. This has been criticized as overly lenient as effective PAP is considered to result in an AHI of $\leq$5 events/h.[39,40] The counterargument is that PAP, although nearly always effective, has suboptimal adherence, and some studies have shown benefit of surgery in terms of mortality and morbidity irrespective of AHI.[41] Four hours of PAP use per night for $\geq$70% of nights meets insurance adherence standards, but this represents less than half the amount of recommended sleep time over the course of a typical week. When incorporating the respiratory events during untreated sleep hours, the effective AHI with such adherence is therefore much higher. Surgically treated patients are by necessity 100% adherent to therapy.

Additional respiratory parameters that may further risk stratify patients include measures of oxygenation, such as the oxygen desaturation index (which measures

Table 4
Severity of obstructive sleep apnea per the apnea-hypopnea index or the respiratory event index

AHI/REI*	Category
<5/h	Normal
5–15/h	Mild
15–30/h	Moderate
>30/h	Severe

Abbreviations: AHI, apnea-hypopnea index; REI, respiratory event index.

* Guidelines do not specify the preferred definition of hypopnea.[13] Although not required by most authorities, logic dictates that different cuts-offs should be applied when the more inclusive definition of hypopnea (ie, allowing events associated with either a >3% desaturation or arousal) is used in contrast to hypopneas limited to those with 4% desaturation. The latter definition is specifically required by the United States Center for Medicare and Medicaid Services in defining eligibility for continuous positive airway pressure. In the former case, the upper limit of "normal" for the AHI may be 10–15/h, and lower limits for mild, moderate, and severe disease may be 20, 35, and 45/h, respectively.

the number of desaturating events of a particular threshold), mean oxygen saturation, nadir oxygen saturation nadir, and total duration of oxygen saturation less than a particular value (90%, for example).[42] Although these parameters are not included in standard severity definitions, they add to the clinical impression of the physiologic implications of the patient's sleep-disordered breathing and are often included as secondary outcome measures in research studies investigating surgical interventions.

Accompanying the quantitative respiratory data should be a qualitative impression of whether the patient displays a tendency toward obstructive or central (or both) phenomena. This is particularly important when most events are unclassified hypopneas. Researchers have analyzed whether the inspiratory flow signal shape during hypopneas can predict the site and type of upper airway obstruction, which could have surgical implications, but this technique remains largely experimental.[43,44] If hypoventilation or Cheyne-Stokes breathing is noted, this should be explicitly stated, as these may alert the reader to other comorbid conditions and preclude upper airway surgery.

PSGs with interventions, particularly ones that are being titrated, such as PAP titrations, report the findings of the interventions. A recommended treatment setting that incorporates the normalization of sleep breathing parameters, patient tolerability, and sleep consolidation, will be stated.

The relation of breathing abnormalities to sleep state and body position is also important, as it can provide diagnostic clues as to the type of sleep-disordered breathing present and have therapeutic implications. Patients with OSA typically show most severe symptoms when supine or in REM sleep, with the combination of the 2 representing the ultimate "OSA stress test." Central sleep apnea, particularly Cheyne-Stokes breathing, on the other hand, is typically less severe in REM. Patients with OSA whose symptoms worsen significantly during supine sleep have supine-predominant or supine-isolated OSA and can be treated with positional therapy.[45] REM-predominant or REM-isolated OSA, although frequently encountered phenotypes, are less amenable to therapeutic interventions, although they may portend prognosis.[46] The amount of REM or sleeping in a particular sleep position is not fixed from night to night, and this may introduce a degree of variability into the patient's AHI dependent solely on contextual factors. Furthermore, it has been suggested that home sleep studies may produce a lower AHI in comparison with PSG in part due to less supine sleep. Variability in the AHI is well documented and is part of the reason that if the clinical suspicion for OSA is high, a repeat PSG should be considered.[13,47–49]

Cardiac

The sleep study report also includes a summary of heart rate data and whether any arrhythmias were noted, particularly if there was any correlation with respiratory events.

Other

Comments on limb movements, EEG phenomenon, such as seizures or alpha intrusion, and observed parasomnias are also reported. A hypnogram, displaying the sleep stages in 30-second epochs for the entire night, is optional but provides an overview of the night's data and is a quick way to correlate sleep architecture with sleep position, respiratory events, or limb movements.

HOME SLEEP APNEA TESTING

Attended PSG aids in the diagnosis of a variety of sleep and nonsleep disorders, including movement disorders, central nervous system hypersomnias, nocturnal seizures, parasomnias, cardiac arrhythmias, gastroesophageal reflux disease, anxiety disorders, and insomnia. Practically, however, the vast majority of PSGs obtained for clinical purposes are related to diagnosing or optimizing treatment of OSA.[50] A diagnosis of OSA can, in the right population, reliably be made with only a fraction of the parameters that are routinely measured on PSG. This, combined with the economic burden and access limitations of widespread PSG testing, has led to the development of less-costly tests that are more accessible to patients.[51] Home sleep apnea testing (HSAT) evolved to fill this need. Other advantages of HSAT, also called out-of-center sleep testing or portable monitoring, include greater convenience to the patient, decreased staffing requirements, and perhaps a more "natural" sleep experience that occurs in the patient's home environment.

Systems for diagnosing OSA traditionally fall into 1 of 4 classifications as defined by the American Sleep Disorders Association (ASDA) guidelines (**Box 3**).[52] Overnight attended PSG classifies as a level I examination and serves as the reference standard. Type II through IV are unattended studies. Types III–IV generally do not include sleep parameters, such as EEG. HSATs most often are level III devices. Most HSATs are done for diagnostic purposes, but they can also be performed to measure the effects

---

Box 3	
Nomenclature of devices used to test for obstructive sleep apnea	
Level I	Attended cardiorespiratory polysomnography with at least 7 signals
Level II	Unattended cardiorespiratory polysomnography with at least 7 signals
Level III	Unattended portable sleep apnea testing with at least 4 signals, including airflow, respiratory effort, oxygen saturation, electrocardiography, or heart rate or pulse rate
Level IV	Unattended portable testing with 1 or 2 signals, such as oximetry and/or heart rate

Data from Mendonça F, Mostafa SS, Ravelo-García AG, Morgado-Dias F, Penzel T. Devices for home detection of obstructive sleep apnea: a review. Sleep Med Rev. 2018;41:149-60.

of interventions, such as oral appliance or positional therapy.[45] HSATs using new technologies, such as those that use peripheral arterial tonometry no longer neatly fit into the ASDA classification.[7] The SCOPER classification system (which incorporates sleep, cardiovascular, oximetry, position, effort and respiratory parameters) was proposed by Collop and colleagues[53] as an alternative and allows for inclusion of these new technologies, but clinical uptake has been slow.

There are several disadvantages of HSAT. Technical failure may occur due to a lack of real-time monitoring of the sensors, which may necessitate repeat testing. This may delay diagnosis and initiation of therapy. Diagnosis of other sleep disorders besides OSA may be overlooked due to the limited parameters recorded and the high prevalence of OSA, which may cause anchoring bias.[51] With home unmonitored testing one loses the opportunity to initiate therapy on the same night in cases of severe OSA, as can be done in a split-night protocol of an attended PSG.[10] Perhaps most importantly, during most HSATs, sleep is not recorded and staged (ie, EEG, EOG, and EMG monitoring are not performed), although some devices use surrogates for EEG (eg, WatchPAT). Many HSATs use recording time instead of sleep time as the denominator when defining respiratory event frequency, which may dilute the calculated frequency of respiratory events in nights when the patient is awake for significant portions. Instead of the AHI, the term respiratory event index (REI) is used for studies without sleep monitoring. REI defines the frequency of apneas and hypopneas per hour of recording time. There is, however, scant literature on cutoffs of REI for OSA disease severity. An additional limitation of HSATs that do not record sleep is that hypopneas can only be defined by oxygen desaturation and hypopneas associated with arousals and RERAs are not measured. Because the hypopneas from an HSAT are defined solely in terms of desaturating events (either 3% or 4%), REI may underestimate the patient's "true" AHI.[7] In the appropriate population, such as severe OSA, the REI and AHI correlate closely. In patients with milder forms of OSA, particularly with concomitant insomnia, the REI may underestimate the AHI considerably. Studies and systematic review data suggest that HSAT using type III devices have false-negative rates of 13% to 20%, and tend to misclassify mostly patients with mild-to-moderate OSA.[51]

Because of these limitations of HSATs, the AASM guidelines recommend PSG as the test of choice for diagnosing OSA, but state that HSAT may be used in the medically uncomplicated adult patient (without cardiopulmonary disease, respiratory muscle weakness, opiate use, history of stroke, and suspected nonrespiratory sleep disorders) presenting with signs and symptoms that indicate an increased risk of moderate to severe OSA. A high pretest probability of moderate to severe OSA is defined as the presence of excessive daytime sleepiness and at least 2 of the following 3 criteria: habitual loud snoring, witnessed apnea or gasping or choking, or diagnosed hypertension. Patients not meeting these criteria should undergo PSG. Furthermore, if HSAT is negative, inconclusive or technically inadequate, most authorities recommend that PSG should be performed as follow-up.[7] PAP after HSAT and PSG using these guidelines have resulted in similar patient-centric outcomes, with a probable cost-advantage. Concerns arise, however, when HSAT is applied inappropriately, either due to incorrect physician referral or misaligned insurance requirements, which may mandate HSAT for all patients, regardless of the pretest probability of OSA.[51] An encouraging recent development is that some newer HSATs incorporate actual or surrogate measures of sleep and arousals in their respiratory event definition (eg, movement, increases in heart rate, or other measures of sympathetic tone).

SUMMARY

This review highlights the important considerations the otorhinolaryngologist must take into account when ordering and interpreting sleep study reports. As the number of patients diagnosed with OSA grows, more will seek out alternative treatment options to CPAP, for whom the otorhinolaryngologist plays a vital role.

DISCLOSURE

The authors have nothing to disclose.

REFERENCES

1. Young T, Palta M, Dempsey J, et al. The occurrence of sleep-disordered breathing among middle-aged adults. N Engl J Med 1993;328(17):1230–5.
2. Young T, Palta M, Dempsey J, et al. Burden of sleep apnea: rationale, design, and major findings of the Wisconsin Sleep Cohort Study. WMJ 2009;108(5):246–9.
3. Veasey SC, Rosen IM. Obstructive sleep apnea in adults. N Engl J Med 2019; 380:1442–9.
4. Peppard PE, Young T, Barnet JH, et al. Increased prevalence of sleep-disordered breathing in adults. Am J Epidemiol 2013;177(9):1006–14.
5. US Preventive Services Task Force, Bibbins-Domingo K, Grossman DC, Curry SJ, et al. Screening for obstructive sleep apnea in adults: US preventive services task force recommendation statement. JAMA 2017;317(4):407–14.
6. Mehra R, Foldvary-Schaefer N. The USPSTF and screening for obstructive sleep apnea: dispelling misconceptions. Cleve Clin J Med 2017;84(6):429–31.
7. Kapur VK, Auckley DH, Chowdhuri S, et al. Clinical practice guideline for diagnostic testing for adult obstructive sleep apnea: an American Academy of Sleep Medicine clinical practice guideline. J Clin Sleep Med 2017;13(3):479–504.
8. Young T, Skatrud J, Peppard PE. Risk factors for obstructive sleep apnea. JAMA 2004;291(16):2013–6.
9. Frey WC, Pilcher J. Obstructive sleep-related breathing disorders in patients evaluated for bariatric surgery. Obes Surg 2003;13(5):676–83.
10. Silber MH. Diagnostic approach and investigation in sleep medicine. Contin (Minneap Minn) 2017;23(4, Sleep Neurology):973–88.
11. Myers KA, Mrkobrada M, Simel DL. Does this patient have obstructive sleep apnea? The rational clinical examination systematic review. JAMA 2013;310(7): 731–41.
12. Lindberg E, Benediktsdottir B, Franklin KA, et al. Women with symptoms of sleep-disordered breathing are less likely to be diagnosed and treated for sleep apnea than men. Sleep Med 2017;35:17–22.
13. Epstein LJ, Kristo D, Strollo PJ, et al. Clinical guideline for the evaluation, management and long-term care of obstructive sleep apnea in adults. J Clin Sleep Med 2009;5(3):263–76.
14. Kohler M, Bloch KE, Stradling JR. The role of the nose in the pathogenesis of obstructive sleep apnea. Curr Opin Otolaryngol Head Neck Surg 2009; 17(1):33–7.
15. Zonato AI, Martinho FL, Bittencourt LR, et al. Head and neck physical examination: comparison between nonapneic and obstructive sleep apnea patients. Laryngoscope 2005;115(6):1030–4.

16. Bolzer A, Toussaint B, Rumeau C, et al. Can anatomical assessment of hypophar-yngolarynx in awake patients predict obstructive sleep apnea? Laryngoscope 2019;129(12):2782–8.
17. Koutsourelakis I, Safiruddin F, Ravesloot M, et al. Surgery for obstructive sleep apnea: sleep endoscopy determinants of outcome. Laryngoscope 2012; 122(11):2587–91.
18. Park D, Kim JS, Heo SJ. Obstruction patterns during drug-induced sleep endos-copy vs natural sleep endoscopy in patients with obstructive sleep apnea. JAMA Otolaryngol Head Neck Surg 2019;145:1–5 [Epub ahead of print].
19. Pang KP, Baptista PM, Olszewska E, et al. Does drug-induced sleep endoscopy affect surgical outcome? A multicenter study of 326 obstructive sleep apnea pa-tients. Laryngoscope 2019;130(2):551–5.
20. Drager LF, Lorenzi-Filho G. POINT: should sleep studies be performed for all pa-tients with poorly controlled hypertension? Yes. Chest 2019;155(6):1095–7.
21. Cardoso CRL, Salles GF. Counterpoint: should sleep studies be performed for all patients with poorly controlled hypertension? No. Chest 2019;155(6):1097–101.
22. Kernan WN, Ovbiagele B, Black HR, et al. Guidelines for the prevention of stroke in patients with stroke and transient ischemic attack. Stroke 2014;45:2160–236.
23. January C, Wann L, Alpert J, et al. 2014 AHA/ACC/HRS guideline for the manage-ment of patients with atrial fibrillation. J Am Coll Cardiol 2014;64(21):e1–76.
24. Berry RB, Wagner MH. Sleep medicine pearls. 3rd edition. Philadelphia: Elsevier Saunders; 2015.
25. Berry RB, Brooks R, Gamaldo CE, et al. The AASM manual for the scoring of sleep and associated events: rules, terminology and technical specifications. Version 2.4. Darien (IL): American Academy of Sleep Medicine; 2017.
26. Redline S, Sanders M. Hypopnea, a floating metric: implications for prevalence, morbidity estimates, and case finding. Sleep 1997;20(12):1209–17.
27. Ayappa I, Norman RG, Krieger AC, et al. Non-invasive detection of respiratory effort-related arousals (RERAs) by a nasal cannula/pressure transducer system. Sleep 2000;23(6):763–71.
28. Pamidi S, Redline S, Rapoport D, et al. An official American Thoracic Society Workshop report: noninvasive identification of inspiratory flow limitation in sleep studies. Ann Am Thorac Soc 2017;14(7):1076–85.
29. Boulos MI, Jairam T, Kendzerska T, et al. Normal polysomnography parameters in healthy adults: a systematic review and meta-analysis. Lancet Respir Med 2019; 7(6):533–43.
30. Malhotra RK, Kirsch DB, Kristo DA, et al. Polysomnography for obstructive sleep apnea should include arousal-based scoring. J Clin Sleep Med 2018;14(7): 1245–7.
31. Stepanski EJ. The effect of sleep fragmentation on daytime function. Sleep 2002; 25(3):268–76.
32. Aldrich M, Chervin R, Malow B. Value of the multiple sleep latency test (MSLT) for the diagnosis of narcolepsy. Sleep 1997;20(8):620–9.
33. American Academy of Sleep Medicine. International classification of sleep disor-ders. 3rd edition. Darien (IL): American Academy of Sleep Medicine; 2014.
34. Redline S, Kapur VK, Sanders MH, et al. Effects of varying approaches for iden-tifying respiratory disturbances on sleep apnea assessment. Am J Respir Crit Care Med 2000;161(2 I):369–74.
35. Duce B, Milosavljevic J, Hukins C. The 2012 AASM respiratory event criteria in-crease the incidence of hypopneas in an adult sleep center population. J Clin Sleep Med 2015;11(12):1425–31.

36. Ruehland WR, Rochford PD, O'Onoghue FJ, et al. The new AASM criteria for scoring hypopneas: impact on the apnea hypopnea index. Sleep 2017;32(2):150–7.

37. Jonas DE, Amick HR, Feltner C, et al. Screening for obstructive sleep apnea in adults evidence report and systematic review for the US preventive services task force. JAMA 2017;317(4):415–33.

38. Kendzerska T, Mollayeva T, Gershon AS, et al. Untreated obstructive sleep apnea and the risk for serious long-term adverse outcomes: a systematic review. Sleep Med Rev 2014;18(1):49–59.

39. Elshaug AG, Moss JR, Southcott AM, et al. Redefining success in airway surgery for obstructive sleep apnea: a meta analysis and synthesis of the evidence. Sleep 2007;30(4):461–7.

40. Caples SM, Rowley JA, Prinsell JR, et al. Surgical modifications of the upper airway for obstructive sleep apnea in adults a systematic review and meta-analysis. Sleep 2010;33(10):1396–407.

41. Lee HM, Kim HY, Suh JD, et al. Uvulopalatopharyngoplasty reduces the incidence of cardiovascular complications caused by obstructive sleep apnea: results from the National Insurance Service Survey 2007–2014. Sleep Med 2018;45:11–6.

42. Kendzerska T, Gershon AS, Hawker G, et al. Obstructive sleep apnea and risk of cardiovascular events and all-cause mortality: a decade-long historical cohort study. PLoS Med 2014;11(2).

43. Aittokallio T, Saaresranta T, Polo-Kantola P, et al. Analysis of inspiratory flow shapes in patients with partial upper-airway obstruction during sleep. Chest 2001;119(1):37–44.

44. Genta PR, Sands SA, Butler JP, et al. Airflow shape is associated with the pharyngeal structure causing OSA. Chest 2017;152(3):537–46.

45. Meliana V, Chung F, Li CK, et al. Interpretation of sleep studies for patients with sleep-disordered breathing: what the anesthesiologist needs to know. Can J Anesth 2018;65(1):60–75.

46. Nisha Aurora R, Crainiceanu C, Gottlieb DJ, et al. Obstructive sleep apnea during REM sleep and cardiovascular disease. Am J Respir Crit Care Med 2018;197(5):653–60.

47. Prasad B, Usmani S, Steffen AD, et al. Short-term variability in apnea-hypopnea index during extended home portable monitoring. J Clin Sleep Med 2016;12(6):855–63.

48. Skiba V, Goldstein C, Schotland H. Night-to-night variability in sleep disordered breathing and the utility of esophageal pressure monitoring in suspected obstructive sleep apnea. J Clin Sleep Med 2015;11(6):597–602.

49. Ahmadi N, Shapiro GK, Chung SA, et al. Clinical diagnosis of sleep apnea based on single night of polysomnography vs. two nights of polysomnography. Sleep Breath 2009;13(3):221–6.

50. Hirshkowitz M. Polysomnography challenges. Sleep Med Clin 2016;11(4):403–11.

51. Rosenberg R, Hirshkowitz M, Rapoport DM, et al. The role of home sleep testing for evaluation of patients with excessive daytime sleepiness: focus on obstructive sleep apnea and narcolepsy. Sleep Med 2019;56:80–9.

52. Mendonça F, Mostafa SS, Ravelo-García AG, et al. Devices for home detection of obstructive sleep apnea: a review. Sleep Med Rev 2018;41:149–60.

53. Collop NA, Tracy SL, Kapur V, et al. Obstructive sleep apnea devices for out-of-center (OOC) testing: technology evaluation. J Clin Sleep Med 2011;7(5):531–48.

The Nose and Nasal Breathing in Sleep Apnea

Yi Cai, MD[a], Andrew N. Goldberg, MD, MS[b], Jolie L. Chang, MD[c],*

KEYWORDS

- Nasal obstruction • Nasal surgery • Nasal sprays • Nasal anatomy
- Obstructive sleep apnea • Sleep-disordered breathing • CPAP compliance
- Sleep outcomes

KEY POINTS

- Assessment of the nose is critical in evaluating obstructive sleep apnea (OSA) because the nose plays an important role in the physiology of sleep by regulating nasal airway resistance and stimulating ventilation.
- Nasal obstruction is common in sleep apnea, contributes to OSA, and interferes with tolerance of OSA treatment with continuous positive airway pressure (CPAP) or oral appliances.
- Medical treatment of nasal obstruction and rhinitis with nasal corticosteroid sprays is associated with improved OSA severity and sleep symptoms.
- Surgery for nasal obstruction, including septoplasty, turbinate reduction, rhinoplasty, and sinus surgery, improves OSA-related quality-of-life measures and CPAP tolerance.
- Patient factors, such as body mass index, tongue position, positional dependency of OSA, and OSA severity, may be influential in predicting OSA improvement after nasal surgery.

NASAL BREATHING IN NORMAL SLEEP

Airflow and resistance in the nasal cavity play important roles in sleep. A normal nose can sustain 20 to 30 L of airflow per minute,[1] and nasal airflow has a stimulant effect on breathing during sleep.[2] Meanwhile, total airway resistance correlates with respiratory effort[3] and in normal subjects, the nasal airway accounts for more than half of the total airway resistance.[4] During sleep, total nasal resistance does not change, although higher nasal resistance levels fluctuate between sides of the nose.[5] Relative changes in nasal resistance between each side of the nose are due to the nasal cycle, a

[a] Department of Otolaryngology–Head and Neck Surgery, University of California, San Francisco, 2233 Post Street, UCSF Box 3213, San Francisco, CA 94115, USA; [b] Department of Otolaryngology–Head and Neck Surgery, University of California, San Francisco, 2233 Post Street, Room 309, San Francisco, CA 94115, USA; [c] Department of Otolaryngology–Head and Neck Surgery, University of California, San Francisco, 2233 Post Street, Box 1225, San Francisco, CA 94115, USA
* Corresponding author.
E-mail address: Jolie.Chang@ucsf.edu

Otolaryngol Clin N Am 53 (2020) 385–395
https://doi.org/10.1016/j.otc.2020.02.002
0030-6665/20/Published by Elsevier Inc.

oto.theclinics.com

physiologic cyclic change in airflow that alternates sides of the nose every 2 to 4 hours.[6] This cycle can be affected by shifts in body position during sleep, with an increase in nasal resistance on the gravity-dependent side of the nose, and a decrease in resistance on the opposite side.[7,8] Airflow through the nose also stimulates a nasal ventilatory reflex with activation of nasal receptors that leads to increased spontaneous ventilation and improved upper-airway muscle tone.[9]

Although the nasal cavity may present a narrow inlet for airflow, nasal breathing is the preferred route for air entry during sleep. Fitzpatrick and colleagues[10] performed a randomized, single-blinded, crossover study of healthy subjects demonstrating a significantly higher apnea-hypopnea index (AHI) (with obstructive and not central events) during oral breathing (43 ± 6) than when compared with nasal breathing (1.5 ± 0.5) during sleep. A few key factors contribute to differences in sleep between the 2 routes of breathing. First, upper-airway resistance during sleep is significantly lower during nasal breathing than during oral breathing (as opposed to equal during the awake state).[10] Next, jaw-opening that occurs during oral breathing in sleep contributes to upper-airway obstruction by decreasing airway patency at the velopharyngeal and tongue-base levels,[11] even in study participants without sleep-disordered breathing (SDB).[12] Lastly, nasal breathing has a stimulating effect on breathing, leading to higher minute ventilation and flow rate[2,13] in addition to greater upper-airway muscle dilation[14] when compared with mouth breathing.

EVALUATION OF NASAL OBSTRUCTION

The external nose is shaped superiorly by paired nasal bones that attach to the nasal process of the maxilla and by two sets of paired cartilages more inferiorly. The upper lateral cartilages define the external middle third of the nose and the lower lateral cartilages, which consist of the medial and lateral crura, define the nasal vestibules or nostrils. Internally, the nose is supported by the nasal septum. There are two nasal valves, which are major regulators of nasal airflow and points of significant airway resistance. Just past the nasal vestibule is the external nasal valve, which is demarcated by the caudal portion of the lower lateral cartilages, columella, and the nasal alar tissue at the pyriform aperture. Further into the nasal cavity, the internal nasal valve is the location of maximum resistance in the nasal cavity and is defined by the lower edge of the upper lateral cartilage, anterior end of the inferior turbinates, and the septum.

Nasal obstruction is defined by the sensation of insufficient airflow through the nose,[15] which can be caused by both inflammatory and structural factors. Common inflammatory diseases causing nasal obstruction include rhinitis, sinusitis, and nasal polyps. Structurally, obstruction can occur at multiple levels. On external examination, the presence of collapse at the nostril (external nasal valve) or lateral nasal wall (internal valve) on inspiration can be determined during natural and forced inspiration to each nostril. Maneuvers such as the modified Cottle maneuver, in which the lateral crus of the lower lateral cartilage (external nasal valve) or the edge of the upper lateral cartilage (internal nasal valve) is supported with a cotton swab or ear curette, help predict whether support of a specific region and nasal valve may improve nasal obstruction.[16] Anterior rhinoscopy is the standard in assessing both anatomic causes and mucosal changes that could be related to nasal obstruction. Anatomically, septal deviation and turbinate hypertrophy are common findings in patients with nasal congestion that have been linked to SDB.[17,18] Although there is no standardized method of grading degree of septal deviation, the inferior turbinate examination can be graded by degree of obstruction of the nasal cavity.[19]

Objective measures of nasal obstruction or resistance are not commonly used during a clinical evaluation but are often reported in research studies. These measures include acoustic rhinometry, imaging, peak inspiratory flow, and computational fluid dynamic analysis.[20] Most clinicians use patient-reported symptoms and patient-reported outcome measures, such as the NOSE score,[21] to assess nasal obstruction severity and change. Studies have attempted to correlate symptom and objective measures of nasal obstruction; however, few have found statistically significant associations. In clinical practice, most treatments focus on optimizing patient-reported symptoms of improved breathing and airflow through the nose.

EVALUATION OF OBSTRUCTIVE SLEEP APNEA

Obstructive sleep apnea (OSA) occurs when repeated reduction or cessation of airflow occurs because of upper-airway collapse during sleep. OSA is associated with symptoms of daytime fatigue, reduced sleep quality, decreased work productivity, increased risk for cardiovascular disease, stroke, and motor-vehicle accidents. The goals of treating sleep apnea are to improve quality of life and reduce health-related risk factors. The severity of OSA is usually graded with the AHI, as measured by polysomnography (PSG), along with oxygen desaturation index (ODI) and respiratory disturbance index (RDI). Just as objective measures of nasal obstruction do not correlate with patient-reported symptoms, AHI value and other measures on the sleep study do not correlate with OSA-related symptom severity scores, quality of life, or symptoms of depression.[22,23]

When selecting treatments for OSA, patient comorbidities, treatment goals, and symptoms must be considered. Nasal symptom query and nasal cavity evaluation are critical components to the complete upper-airway evaluation in sleep apnea. Standard first-line medical therapy for OSA includes positive airway pressure (PAP), which includes continuous positive airway pressure (CPAP), autoadjusting PAP, and bilevel PAP with a variety of mask interface options. For many patients, the nasal pillow–PAP interface can be the easiest to manage. For patients who fail PAP therapy, other treatment modalities such as an oral appliance, behavioral treatments, or surgery are considered. Surgical success is traditionally defined in the literature as a greater than 50% reduction in AHI and a final AHI of less than 20. However, overall disease burden reduction drives symptom improvements, and it is beneficial to consider multimodality and staged treatment approaches for sleep apnea.[24]

NASAL OBSTRUCTION IN SLEEP APNEA

Nasal obstruction is a common comorbidity in OSA. A recent study of 810 patients in the Icelandic Sleep Apnea Cohort showed that nocturnal nasal congestion occurs at least once per week in 65% of treatment-naïve OSA patients and at least three times a week in 35% of patients.[25] Similarly, a study of more than 2600 adult patients who underwent in-laboratory PSG showed that 65% of patients experienced nasal obstruction symptoms.[26]

In the physiologic Starling resistor model of OSA, the nose is regarded as a fixed and constricted inlet that affects downstream collapse of the oropharynx and hypopharynx.[27-29] According to this model, when air is drawn through a narrowed inlet at the nose, a negative intraluminal pressure is generated downstream in the collapsible segment of the upper airway at the oropharynx and hypopharynx that can result in pharyngeal collapse and apnea. Theoretically, with this simplified model, relief of significant obstruction at the nasal inlet of the airway can reduce the negative pressures that contribute to OSA. In reality, other factors, such as anatomy of the oropharynx, tongue, hypopharynx, and jaw structure, play important roles in the upper-airway collapse of OSA. Ventilatory control, resting muscle tone, and arousal thresholds are also vital components of disease pathophysiology.

Nasal obstruction may also contribute to or exacerbate OSA. In a study of OSA patients who underwent nasal surgery, postoperative nasal packing (iatrogenically inducing complete nasal obstruction) increased the RDI, duration of snoring, and ODI in patients with mild but not moderate to severe OSA.[30] Studies have shown a positive correlation between nasal obstruction (as measured by acoustic rhinometry) and RDI in nonobese patients[31] and an inverse correlation between nasal volume and AHI as well as ODI.[32] Furthermore, total nasal resistance in nonobese patients has been shown to correlate with AHI in the supine position, but not in the seated position.[32] Large-scale population studies also suggest nasal obstruction is an independent contributor to OSA. Survey results of 4927 subjects showed a significant association between frequent nighttime nasal congestion and habitual snoring, chronic daytime sleepiness, and chronic nonrestorative sleep.[33] In the Icelandic Sleep Apnea Cohort, nocturnal nasal obstruction was significantly associated with increased daytime sleepiness and reduced mental health quality-of-life scores.[25] Thus, nasal obstruction plays a role in recurrent airway collapse during sleep by affecting snoring, daytime sleepiness, AHI, RDI, and ODI. Also of note, the impact of nasal obstruction on sleep-related metrics and quality-of-life measures may be more pronounced in nonobese patients with mild to moderate positional sleep apnea.

Common structural causes of nasal obstruction in OSA include septal deviation, turbinate hypertrophy and maxillary narrowing. A study of 67 patients with either habitual snoring or OSA–hypopnea syndrome found evidence of inferior turbinate hypertrophy in 97% of the patients and increased nasal resistance on acoustic rhinometry in 93% of patients.[18] Similarly, a study of 293 OSA patients found that 85% of the patients with nasal obstruction (which was present in 64% of the sample) had septal deviation and/or turbinate hypertrophy.[34] In comparison, a study of 100 non-OSA patients demonstrated the prevalence of significant septal deviation and turbinate hypertrophy was much lower at 1% and 31%, respectively.[35]

Beyond anatomic causes of nasal obstruction, changes to the nasal mucosa, such as edema from rhinitis or polyps associated with chronic rhinosinusitis (CRS), may contribute to nasal obstruction. Nonallergic rhinitis (NAR) is more common[26] and has been associated with a greater risk of OSA when compared with allergic rhinitis (AR). In a study of age- and sex-matched AR (confirmed by skin prick testing) and NAR patients who underwent PSG, OSA syndrome was diagnosed in 83% of NAR patients, compared with in 36% of AR patients.[36] Meanwhile, CRS is a less frequent comorbid condition in OSA patients. In an analysis of the Taiwan Longitudinal Health Insurance Database, the 5-year incidence of CRS was 6.6% in OSA patients and 2.0% in patients without OSA.[37] However, CRS is an important entity to consider in OSA patients with nasal obstruction because more than 75% of patients with CRS report abnormal sleep quality[38] and PSG-confirmed OSA has been found in up to 65% of CRS patients undergoing surgery.[39] Furthermore, a recently published study of World Trade Center responders concluded that CRS is an independent risk factor for OSA (odds ratio of 1.80; $P = .006$), even after adjusting for age, body mass index (BMI), sex, gastroesophageal reflux disorder, and alcohol use.[40] Although the precise pathophysiologic mechanism of the relationship between CRS and sleep changes is not yet fully understood, theories range from CRS-associated nasal obstruction owing to mucosal edema and inflammatory polypoid disease to inflammatory cytokine release in allergy-mediated disease that influences the sleep/wake cycle directly.[41]

Nasal obstruction can also play an important role in the tolerance of treatment modalities for OSA. In a study of 77 OSA patients who received CPAP with nasal masks, higher nasal resistance on rhinomanometry was found to be a statistically significant predictor of CPAP noncompliance.[42] Furthermore, a study of 13 CPAP-tolerant and 12 CPAP-intolerant patients with similar average age, gender, CPAP level, BMI, and RDI showed a greater cross-sectional area of the inferior turbinates in the CPAP-intolerant group.[43] Nasal obstruction can also interfere with oral appliance treatment of OSA. In a study of 38 OSA patients who were treated with an oral appliance, nasal airway resistance was increased in the group of 12 nonresponders when compared with oral appliance responders. On logistic regression analysis, nasal airway resistance was identified as one of the most important predictive factors of oral appliance response.[44]

MEDICAL TREATMENTS FOR NASAL OBSTRUCTION IN OBSTRUCTIVE SLEEP APNEA

The most frequently used medications for nasal obstruction in OSA are topical nasal steroid sprays, which have been shown to improve sleep outcomes. In a randomized, placebo-controlled, crossover study of OSA patients with rhinitis, median AHI was significantly lower following 4 weeks' treatment with intranasal fluticasone when compared with placebo (23.3 vs 30.3; $P<.05$).[45] Similarly, OSA patients with AR had significantly improved lowest oxygen saturation (LSAT) and supine AHI after 10 to 12 weeks' treatment with intranasal corticosteroids.[46] Furthermore, AR patients with sleep-related complaints treated with intranasal corticosteroids reported significant improvement in subjective sleep.[47]

Efficacy of internal nasal dilators and external dilator strips for nasal obstruction in those with OSA is equivocal. External nasal dilators have been shown to have beneficial effects on subjective snoring but mixed results in effects on frequency of apneas or daytime sleepiness.[48] For instance, use of a plastic external nasal dilator in a small group of patients with snoring or OSA resulted in statistically significant improvements in the apnea index (from a mean of 18 to 6.4) and snoring noise but did not affect daytime hypersomnolence.[49] Similarly, in a randomized, placebo- and sham-controlled crossover study of OSA patients with nasal obstruction treated with a topical decongestant and external dilator strip, AHI decreased by an average of 12/h ($P<.02$), and RDI improved from an average of 40 to 30 events/h ($P = .02$) in the treatment group, but there were no changes in sleepiness scores.[50] In contrast, a double-blind, randomized controlled crossover study in patients with upper-airway resistance syndrome did not show a change in AHI with nasal dilator use, although stage 1 sleep and overall desaturation time both decreased.[51] In a 2016 metaanalysis of 14 studies of nasal dilator use in a total of 147 OSA patients, there were no significant changes in AHI or LSAT with internal or external nasal dilator use.[52] However, there was a small reduction in apnea index (by 4.9 events/h) with internal nasal dilator use.[52]

SURGICAL TREATMENTS FOR NASAL OBSTRUCTION IN OBSTRUCTIVE SLEEP APNEA

Various surgical treatments for nasal obstruction, including inferior turbinate reduction, septoplasty, rhinoplasty for nasal valve repair, and functional endoscopic sinus surgery, have been studied in the context of OSA treatment. PSG data, such as AHI, RDI, and LSAT, as well as sleep symptom scores, such as the Epworth sleepiness scale (ESS),[53] are the most commonly reported metrics used in assessing efficacy of these interventions. Individual studies have shown an improvement in AHI after nasal surgeries,[54] including functional septorhinoplasty,[55] endoscopic sinus surgery,[56] and septoplasty with inferior turbinate reduction[57] for nasal obstruction. Most surgical studies have been small, non-randomized trials. Although past metaanalyses on the topic found no change in AHI after nasal surgery,[58,59] the more recent systematic review and metaanalysis by Wu and colleagues[54] in 2017 found a statistically significant, but small decrease in AHI following isolated nasal surgery. In this analysis, 17 studies met inclusion criteria of investigating isolated nasal surgery in adults with preoperative and postoperative quantitative data evaluating at least AHI and ESS.[54] They found a statistically significant improvement in AHI of −4.15 with a 95% confidence interval (CI) of −6.48 to −1.82 after surgery. Subgroup analysis also showed statistically significant reductions in both AHI and ESS after isolated nasal surgery.[54] Wu and colleagues cite the increased number of studies as a reason for differing conclusions regarding AHI when compared with the 2015 meta-analysis by Ishii and colleagues of 10 studies performed using similar systematic review methods and inclusion criteria. Although no significant AHI change was found, Ishii and colleagues[58] did show a significant improvement in average RDI of −11.06 (95% CI of −16.19 to −5.92) after surgery. Of note, there is notable heterogeneity among the small studies on nasal surgery with inconsistency in patient selection criteria for surgery and inconsistent evaluation of OSA. Small sample sizes and relatively short follow-up periods in these studies also limit the interpretation and generalizability of the findings. Overall, nasal surgery for nasal obstruction in OSA appears to provide a small to moderate improvement in AHI and RDI. The discrepancies within the current literature suggest a subgroup or particular phenotype of certain OSA patients may exhibit a larger impact on AHI improvement, although the criteria for this subgroup needs to be better defined.

While the effect of nasal surgery in OSA on AHI may be debated, there is a consensus on the impact of nasal surgery on improved sleep symptoms and daytime fatigue after surgery. In their meta-analyses, Wu and colleagues[54] found a change in ESS of −4.08 (95% CI of −5.27 to −2.88) after nasal surgery, and Ishii and colleagues[58] found a change in ESS of −3.53 (95% CI of −6.23 to −0.64). Even in a subgroup of OSA patients who did not experience changes in their AHI or RDI after nasal surgery (termed "nonresponders"), Park and colleagues[60] found that these patients still experienced significant improvements in daytime somnolence and rapid eye movement sleep time. Thus, nasal surgery can improve patient-reported measures of daytime fatigue.

Body weight and Friedman tongue position[61] may be important factors in predicting response to nasal surgery in sleep apnea patients. In a study of 44 SDB patients, nasal obstruction (measured by acoustic rhinometry) correlated more strongly with RDI in nonobese subjects than in the overall sample.[31] Furthermore, Li and colleagues found that lower BMI and lower Friedman tongue position were associated with significantly higher success rates with improved Snore Outcome Survey and ESS scores after nasal surgery.[62]

Position-dependent OSA may also be a positive predictor of response to surgery for nasal obstruction in OSA patients. In a study of 79 OSA patients with nasal obstruction, when results were analyzed by OSA severity alone, only mild OSA patients were found to have statistically significant improvements in AHI, LSAT, supine AHI, and arousal indexes after nasal surgery.[63] However, with subgroup analysis by positional dependency of OSA, patients with moderate positional OSA were also found to have a statistically significant increase in LSAT and decrease in AHI.[63] These findings are consistent with the theory that nasal obstruction may have a more important role in mild to moderate sleep apnea, whereas other areas of upper-airway collapse are more significant factors in more severe disease. Thus, the ability for nasal surgery to cure or resolve OSA is not universal but may be beneficial for certain patient subgroups, such as those who are nonobese with positional OSA.

Nasal surgery can also play an important role in improving CPAP compliance because nasal congestion is a commonly reported factor in CPAP intolerance.[64] In a systematic review and meta-analysis of patients with OSA and nasal obstruction, nasal surgery was shown to reduce average therapeutic CPAP pressures from 11.6 ± 2.2 cm H_2O to 9.5 ± 2.0 cm H_2O and 89.1% of patients who were not using CPAP before nasal surgery subsequently adhered to or tolerated it.[65] In addition, in a study of 12 CPAP-intolerant patients with severe OSA syndrome who underwent surgery for nasal obstruction, all became tolerant to CPAP; ESS scores decreased from 11.7 to 3.3 ($P<.05$), and LSAT increased from 68% to 75% ($P<.05$), though the AHI did not change.[66] Furthermore, in a cost-analysis study, nasal surgery was shown to be a cost-effective method of improving CPAP compliance among nonadherent CPAP users.[67]

DISCUSSION

Although often underestimated, the nose plays an important role in OSA and nasal obstruction negatively affects sleep quality and OSA severity. Nasal evaluation and nasal obstruction management are a crucial part of comprehensive OSA treatment. In OSA patients with nasal obstruction, medical treatment has shown efficacy in those with rhinitis. Structural causes of nasal obstruction include septal deviation, turbinate hypertrophy, or nasal valve collapse. Given the high prevalence of rhinitis and nasal obstruction in OSA, it is reasonable and recommended to initiate a trial of medical therapy in patients with nasal obstruction. If medical therapy is not efficacious or well tolerated, nasal surgery can improve sleep quality, daytime fatigue, and measures of OSA severity. Moreover, nasal obstruction treatments also enhance PAP tolerance and may improve oral appliance management in OSA.

Despite an emphasis on AHI and PSG metrics in measurements of OSA treatment response, improvement in subjective symptoms of OSA, such as daytime fatigue and measures of sleep-related quality of life, should not be overlooked. Existing pooled analyses have shown mixed results in AHI change after nasal surgery in OSA patients, but consistently demonstrated improved sleep symptoms, quality of life, and PAP tolerance.

Defining a nasal obstruction–predominant OSA phenotype may assist in selecting and counseling patients about the benefits of nasal surgery. Certain subgroups of OSA patients may be more likely to benefit from nasal obstruction management than others. Nonobese BMI, lower Friedman tongue position, positional dependence of OSA, and baseline mild OSA are potential predictors of improved sleep apnea metrics after nasal surgery. An and colleagues[68] conducted a recent randomized, placebo-controlled, double-blind crossover trial of 15 OSA patients with nasal obstruction-predominant disease (defined by nasal obstruction symptoms with corresponding endoscopic findings, lower Friedman tongue position, and lack of tonsillar hypertrophy). Nasal decongestion with oxymetazoline in this group correlated with a statistically significant improvement in sleep quality, total AHI, supine AHI, and ODI during sleep when compared with placebo nasal saline sprays. Nasal obstruction-predominant OSA could also be defined by degree of oral breathing during sleep. A study by Koutsourelakis and colleagues[69] showed that patients with the lowest baseline nasal breathing epochs and those who had the largest improvement in nasal breathing epochs after nasal surgery were the ones with the most significant reduction in AHI. This finding suggests that successful conversion from oral to nasal breathing during sleep is important. Certainly, further research is needed to identify OSA patients with nasal obstruction who would most benefit from nasal obstruction management.

SUMMARY

Effective treatment of the nasal airway is vital to the complete management of the upper airway in sleep apnea. Nasal obstruction is associated with reduced sleep quality, increased daytime fatigue, and an increased risk of snoring and OSA. Chronic obstruction negatively affects PAP and oral appliance tolerance. Medical management of nasal congestion has a role in the context of rhinitis in OSA. For those who fail medical therapy, surgery to improve nasal airway patency can improve sleep quality, snoring, and daytime fatigue. Nasal surgery alone has a small effect in lowering the AHI, the most common objective measure of sleep apnea severity. However, nasal surgery for obstruction has been shown to improve sleep-related quality-of-life measures and can alter sleep architecture and breathing in sleep. Improved nasal airway patency can also lower PAP pressure requirements and improve adherence in patients who report limited PAP use and concurrent nasal obstruction. Further understanding of the predictors for significant sleep apnea benefit with nasal obstruction management is required.

DISCLOSURE

A.N. Goldberg is a consultant and minor stockholder in Keyssa, Inc and Siesta Medical as well as an inventor on a pending sinus diagnostics and therapeutics patent. The terms of this arrangement have been reviewed and approved by the University of California, San Francisco in accordance with its policy on objectivity in research. The other authors have nothing to disclose.

REFERENCES

1. Sahin-Yilmaz A, Naclerio RM. Anatomy and physiology of the upper airway. Proc Am Thorac Soc 2011;8(1):31–9.
2. McNicholas WT, Coffey M, Boyle T. Effects of nasal airflow on breathing during sleep in normal humans. Am Rev Respir Dis 1993;147(3):620–3.
3. Lopes JM, Tabachnik E, Muller NL, et al. Total airway resistance and respiratory muscle activity during sleep. J Appl Physiol Respir Environ Exerc Physiol 1983; 54(3):773–7.
4. Ferris BG Jr, Mead J, Opie LH. Partitioning of respiratory flow resistance in man. J Appl Physiol 1964;19:653–8.
5. Hudgel DW, Robertson DW. Nasal resistance during wakefulness and sleep in normal man. Acta Otolaryngol 1984;98(1–2):130–5.
6. Lang C, Grutzenmacher S, Mlynski B, et al. Investigating the nasal cycle using endoscopy, rhinoresistometry, and acoustic rhinometry. Laryngoscope 2003; 113(2):284–9.
7. Rao S, Potdar A. Nasal airflow with body in various positions. J Appl Physiol 1970; 28(2):162–5.
8. Rohrmeier C, Schittek S, Ettl T, et al. The nasal cycle during wakefulness and sleep and its relation to body position. Laryngoscope 2014;124(6):1492–7.
9. Baraniuk JN, Merck SJ. Nasal reflexes: implications for exercise, breathing, and sex. Curr Allergy Asthma Rep 2008;8(2):147–53.
10. Fitzpatrick MF, McLean H, Urton AM, et al. Effect of nasal or oral breathing route on upper airway resistance during sleep. Eur Respir J 2003;22(5):827–32.
11. Virkkula P, Hurmerinta K, Loytonen M, et al. Postural cephalometric analysis and nasal resistance in sleep-disordered breathing. Laryngoscope 2003;113(7): 1166–74.

12. Meurice JC, Marc I, Carrier G, et al. Effects of mouth opening on upper airway collapsibility in normal sleeping subjects. Am J Respir Crit Care Med 1996; 153(1):255–9.

13. Douglas NJ, White DP, Weil JV, et al. Effect of breathing route on ventilation and ventilatory drive. Respir Physiol 1983;51(2):209–18.

14. Basner RC, Simon PM, Schwartzstein RM, et al. Breathing route influences upper airway muscle activity in awake normal adults. J Appl Physiol (1985) 1989;66(4): 1766–71.

15. Jessen M, Malm L. Definition, prevalence and development of nasal obstruction. Allergy 1997;52(40 Suppl):3–6.

16. Fung E, Hong P, Moore C, et al. The effectiveness of modified Cottle maneuver in predicting outcomes in functional rhinoplasty. Plast Surg Int 2014;2014:618313.

17. Silvoniemi P, Suonpaa J, Sipila J, et al. Sleep disorders in patients with severe nasal obstruction due to septal deviation. Acta Otolaryngol Suppl 1997;529: 199–201.

18. Lenders H, Schaefer J, Pirsig W. Turbinate hypertrophy in habitual snorers and patients with obstructive sleep apnea: findings of acoustic rhinometry. Laryngoscope 1991;101(6 Pt 1):614–8.

19. Camacho M, Zaghi S, Certal V, et al. Inferior turbinate classification system, grades 1 to 4: development and validation study. Laryngoscope 2015;125(2): 296–302.

20. Spataro E, Most SP. Measuring nasal obstruction outcomes. Otolaryngol Clin North Am 2018;51(5):883–95.

21. Stewart MG, Witsell DL, Smith TL, et al. Development and validation of the Nasal Obstruction Symptom Evaluation (NOSE) scale. Otolaryngol Head Neck Surg 2004;130(2):157–63.

22. Macey PM, Woo MA, Kumar R, et al. Relationship between obstructive sleep apnea severity and sleep, depression and anxiety symptoms in newly-diagnosed patients. PLoS One 2010;5(4):e10211.

23. Weaver EM, Woodson BT, Steward DL. Polysomnography indexes are discordant with quality of life, symptoms, and reaction times in sleep apnea patients. Otolaryngol Head Neck Surg 2005;132(2):255–62.

24. Holty JE, Guilleminault C. Surgical options for the treatment of obstructive sleep apnea. Med Clin North Am 2010;94(3):479–515.

25. Varendh M, Andersson M, Bjornsdottir E, et al. Nocturnal nasal obstruction is frequent and reduces sleep quality in patients with obstructive sleep apnea. J Sleep Res 2018;27(4):e12631.

26. Krakow B, Foley-Shea M, Ulibarri VA, et al. Prevalence of potential nonallergic rhinitis at a community-based sleep medical center. Sleep Breath 2016;20(3): 987–93.

27. Park SS. Flow-regulatory function of upper airway in health and disease: a unified pathogenetic view of sleep-disordered breathing. Lung 1993;171(6):311–33.

28. Schwartz AR, Smith PL, Wise RA, et al. Induction of upper airway occlusion in sleeping individuals with subatmospheric nasal pressure. J Appl Physiol (1985) 1988;64(2):535–42.

29. Smith PL, Wise RA, Gold AR, et al. Upper airway pressure-flow relationships in obstructive sleep apnea. J Appl Physiol (1985) 1988;64(2):789–95.

30. Friedman M, Maley A, Kelley K, et al. Impact of nasal obstruction on obstructive sleep apnea. Otolaryngol Head Neck Surg 2011;144(6):1000–4.

31. Morris LG, Burschtin O, Lebowitz RA, et al. Nasal obstruction and sleep-disordered breathing: a study using acoustic rhinometry. Am J Rhinol 2005; 19(1):33–9.
32. Virkkula P, Maasilta P, Hytönen M, et al. Nasal obstruction and sleep-disordered breathing: the effect of supine body position on nasal measurements in snorers. Acta Otolaryngol 2009;123(5):648–54.
33. Young T, Finn L, Kim H. Nasal obstruction as a risk factor for sleep-disordered breathing. The University of Wisconsin Sleep and Respiratory Research Group. J Allergy Clin Immunol 1997;99(2):S757–62.
34. Zonato AI, Bittencourt LR, Martinho FL, et al. Association of systematic head and neck physical examination with severity of obstructive sleep apnea-hypopnea syndrome. Laryngoscope 2003;113(6):973–80.
35. Zonato AI, Martinho FL, Bittencourt LR, et al. Head and neck physical examination: comparison between nonapneic and obstructive sleep apnea patients. Laryngoscope 2005;115(6):1030–4.
36. Kalpaklioglu AF, Kavut AB, Ekici M. Allergic and nonallergic rhinitis: the threat for obstructive sleep apnea. Ann Allergy Asthma Immunol 2009;103(1):20–5.
37. Kao LT, Hung SH, Lin HC, et al. Obstructive sleep apnea and the subsequent risk of chronic rhinosinusitis: a population-based study. Sci Rep 2016;6:20786.
38. Alt JA, Smith TL, Mace JC, et al. Sleep quality and disease severity in patients with chronic rhinosinusitis. Laryngoscope 2013;123(10):2364–70.
39. Jiang RS, Liang KL, Hsin CH, et al. The impact of chronic rhinosinusitis on sleep-disordered breathing. Rhinology 2016;54(1):75–9.
40. Sunderram J, Weintraub M, Black K, et al. Chronic rhinosinusitis is an independent risk factor for OSA in World Trade Center responders. Chest 2019;155(2): 375–83.
41. Alt JA, Smith TL. Chronic rhinosinusitis and sleep: a contemporary review. Int Forum Allergy Rhinol 2013;3(11):941–9.
42. Sugiura T, Noda A, Nakata S, et al. Influence of nasal resistance on initial acceptance of continuous positive airway pressure in treatment for obstructive sleep apnea syndrome. Respiration 2007;74(1):56–60.
43. Morris LG, Setlur J, Burschtin OE, et al. Acoustic rhinometry predicts tolerance of nasal continuous positive airway pressure: a pilot study. Am J Rhinol 2006;20(2): 133–7.
44. Zeng B, Ng AT, Qian J, et al. Influence of nasal resistance on oral appliance treatment outcome in obstructive sleep apnea. Sleep 2008;31(4):543–7.
45. Kiely JL, Nolan P, McNicholas WT. Intranasal corticosteroid therapy for obstructive sleep apnoea in patients with co-existing rhinitis. Thorax 2004;59(1):50–5.
46. Lavigne F, Petrof BJ, Johnson JR, et al. Effect of topical corticosteroids on allergic airway inflammation and disease severity in obstructive sleep apnoea. Clin Exp Allergy 2013;43(10):1124–33.
47. Craig TJ, Teets S, Lehman EB, et al. Nasal congestion secondary to allergic rhinitis as a cause of sleep disturbance and daytime fatigue and the response to topical nasal corticosteroids. J Allergy Clin Immunol 1998;101(5):633–7.
48. Kohler M, Bloch KE, Stradling JR. The role of the nose in the pathogenesis of obstructive sleep apnoea and snoring. Eur Respir J 2007;30(6):1208–15.
49. Hoijer U, Ejnell H, Hedner J, et al. The effects of nasal dilation on snoring and obstructive sleep apnea. Arch Otolaryngol Head Neck Surg 1992;118(3):281–4.
50. McLean HA, Urton AM, Driver HS, et al. Effect of treating severe nasal obstruction on the severity of obstructive sleep apnoea. Eur Respir J 2005;25(3):521–7.

51. Bahammam AS, Tate R, Manfreda J, et al. Upper airway resistance syndrome: effect of nasal dilation, sleep stage, and sleep position. Sleep 1999;22(5):592–8.
52. Camacho M, Malu OO, Kram YA, et al. Nasal dilators (Breathe Right Strips and NoZovent) for snoring and OSA: a systematic review and meta-analysis. Pulm Med 2016;2016:4841310.
53. Johns MW. A new method for measuring daytime sleepiness: the Epworth sleepiness scale. Sleep 1991;14(6):540–5.
54. Wu J, Zhao G, Li Y, et al. Apnea-hypopnea index decreased significantly after nasal surgery for obstructive sleep apnea: a meta-analysis. Medicine (Baltimore) 2017;96(5):e6008.
55. Shuaib SW, Undavia S, Lin J, et al. Can functional septorhinoplasty independently treat obstructive sleep apnea? Plast Reconstr Surg 2015;135(6):1554–65.
56. Yalamanchali S, Cipta S, Waxman J, et al. Effects of endoscopic sinus surgery and nasal surgery in patients with obstructive sleep apnea. Otolaryngol Head Neck Surg 2014;151(1):171–5.
57. Moxness MH, Nordgard S. An observational cohort study of the effects of septoplasty with or without inferior turbinate reduction in patients with obstructive sleep apnea. BMC Ear Nose Throat Disord 2014;14:11.
58. Ishii L, Roxbury C, Godoy A, et al. Does nasal surgery improve OSA in patients with nasal obstruction and OSA? A meta-analysis. Otolaryngol Head Neck Surg 2015;153(3):326–33.
59. Li HY, Wang PC, Chen YP, et al. Critical appraisal and meta-analysis of nasal surgery for obstructive sleep apnea. Am J Rhinol Allergy 2011;25(1):45–9.
60. Park CY, Hong JH, Lee JH, et al. Clinical effect of surgical correction for nasal pathology on the treatment of obstructive sleep apnea syndrome. PLoS One 2014; 9(6):e98765.
61. Friedman M, Ibrahim H, Bass L. Clinical staging for sleep-disordered breathing. Otolaryngol Head Neck Surg 2002;127(1):13–21.
62. Li HY, Lee LA, Wang PC, et al. Can nasal surgery improve obstructive sleep apnea: subjective or objective? Am J Rhinol Allergy 2009;23(6):e51–5.
63. Hu B, Han D, Li Y, et al. Polysomnographic effect of nasal surgery on positional and non-positional obstructive sleep apnea/hypopnea patients. Acta Otolaryngol 2013;133(8):858–65.
64. Hoffstein V, Viner S, Mateika S, et al. Treatment of obstructive sleep apnea with nasal continuous positive airway pressure. Patient compliance, perception of benefits, and side effects. Am Rev Respir Dis 1992;145(4 Pt 1):841–5.
65. Camacho M, Riaz M, Capasso R, et al. The effect of nasal surgery on continuous positive airway pressure device use and therapeutic treatment pressures: a systematic review and meta-analysis. Sleep 2015;38(2):279–86.
66. Nakata S, Noda A, Yagi H, et al. Nasal resistance for determinant factor of nasal surgery in CPAP failure patients with obstructive sleep apnea syndrome. Rhinology 2005;43(4):296–9.
67. Kempfle JS, BuSaba NY, Dobrowski JM, et al. A cost-effectiveness analysis of nasal surgery to increase continuous positive airway pressure adherence in sleep apnea patients with nasal obstruction. Laryngoscope 2017;127(4):977–83.
68. An Y, Li Y, Kang D, et al. The effects of nasal decongestion on obstructive sleep apnoea. Am J Otolaryngol 2019;40(1):52–6.
69. Koutsourelakis I, Georgoulopoulos G, Perraki E, et al. Randomised trial of nasal surgery for fixed nasal obstruction in obstructive sleep apnoea. Eur Respir J 2008;31(1):110–7.

Oral Appliances for Snoring and Obstructive Sleep Apnea

Samuel A. Mickelson, MD, FACS, FABSM

KEYWORDS

- Sleep oral appliance • Mandibular advancement device (MAD)
- Oral appliance therapy (OAT) • Primary snoring • Obstructive sleep apnea syndrome
- OSAS

KEY POINTS

- The efficacy of a mandibular advancement device is less than that of continuous positive airway pressure (CPAP) but mandibular advancement devices have similar effectiveness, with a self-reported compliance rate of approximately 80%, and typically are preferred over CPAP.
- Due to improved compliance, mandibular advancement devices are reasonable second-line treatments of patients who refuse or fail positive airway pressure (PAP) and potentially first-line treatment options.
- Mandibular advancement devices are effective in reducing apnea-hypopnea index via a nonlinear dose-dependent relationship with degree of advancement, and greater protrusion often results in better outcomes.
- Relative contraindications for a mandibular advancement device include loose teeth, significant dental carries or periodontitis, severe bruxism, upcoming dental work or braces, temporomandibular joint (TMJ) pain, significant nasal obstruction, and findings of TMJ crepitation or popping, or inadequate mandibular protrusion.
- Side effects of mandibular advancement devices are common but typically can be managed by slowing protrusion of the appliance. TMJ or dental pain is the most common problem associated with these appliances followed by occlusal changes and shifting of the teeth.

OVERVIEW AND HISTORY OF ORAL APPLIANCE THERAPY

The first mandibular advancement type of oral appliance for sleep apnea was developed in 1988, designed as maxillary boil-and-bite fixed appliance with a plastic extension behind the mandibular incisors and intended to protrude the mandible by pressing on the mandibular incisors. The appliance was soon found to cause anterior displacement of the mandibular incisors and also had problems with retention on the

Advanced Ear, Nose & Throat Associates, The Atlanta Snoring and Sleep Disorders Institute, 960 Johnson Ferry Road NE, Suite 200, Atlanta, GA 30342, USA
E-mail address: samm4028@gmail.com

Otolaryngol Clin N Am 53 (2020) 397–407
https://doi.org/10.1016/j.otc.2020.02.004
0030-6665/20/© 2020 Elsevier Inc. All rights reserved.

maxillary dentition. In 1992, the appliance was modified to be a fixed-position mandibular and maxillary appliance, allowing better protrusion of the mandible. The dental retention problem persisted, however, due to the boil-and-bite technology, and patients began having temporomandibular joint (TMJ) pain and stiffness after wearing the appliance, because the appliance did not allow any lateral motion.

The first custom-made, adjustable mandibular advancement device (MAD) was developed in 1994, requiring full dental impressions, stone models, and a bite registration. The thermoactive acrylic appliance had attached Adams ball clasps (Klearway appliance, Great Lakes Dental Technologies, Tonawanda, NY [Fig. 1]) and allowed much better retention than the boil-and-bite devices. Its design also allowed for lateral motion during sleep, causing much less TMJ pain and stiffness in the morning, and the device was adjustable to allow a slow protrusion of up to 11 mm of the mandible. Since then, hundreds of mandibular advancement devices have been developed with a variety of materials (see Fig. 1).

A tongue-retaining device (TRD) was the first sleep oral appliance, developed in 1982, designed as a soft plastic bulb that was squeezed before inserting the tongue into it. The bulb creates a suction that holds the tongue out of the mouth and protrudes the base of tongue during sleep. Currently, TRDs are used rarely but are available from a variety of sources on the Internet and are available to patients in the United States without a prescription. TRDs have a lower compliance rate than MADs,[1,2] often due to tongue irritation, and there are few published data on efficacy.

MECHANISM OF ACTION OF SLEEP ORAL APPLIANCES

MADs work by advancing the mandible and base of tongue, resulting in traction on the lateral pharyngeal walls and potentially tensioning of the genioglossus and geniohyoid

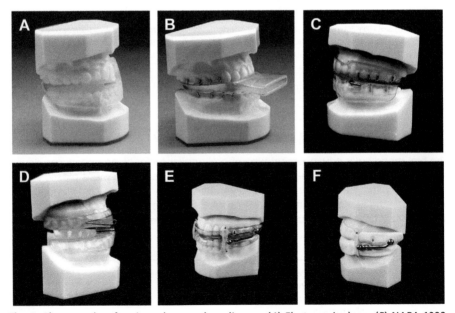

Fig. 1. Photographs of various sleep oral appliances. (A) Elastomeric sleep, (B) NAPA 1000, (C) Klearway, (D) dreamTAP, (E) hard Telescopic Sleep Herbst, and (F) soft Telescopic Sleep Herbst. (Photos provided by Great Lakes Dental Technologies, Tonawanda, NY.)

muscles. In theory, the more advancement of the mandible, the greater the improvement should be on the pharyngeal airway. Endoscopy and magnetic resonance imaging studies have shown primarily retropalatal airway enlargement,[3,4] likely caused by tensioning of the genioglossus muscle, palatoglossus muscles, and anterior positioning of the mandibular ramus with the associated pharyngeal soft tissues. The airway is enlarged more in the lateral pharyngeal walls, likely due to traction of the mandibular ramus.[5] Wearing a mandibular advancement device that is not advanced beyond centric occlusion has been shown to have no effect on airway size or sleep apnea[6] whereas efficacy is correlated to the degree of mandibular advancement.[7–9]

PATIENT SELECTION, REQUIREMENTS, AND LIMITATIONS

To wear a mandibular advancement sleep oral appliance, a patient must have sufficient stable dentition: typically 6 teeth to 8 teeth per arch. If fewer than these exist in any arch, then the appliance may cause significant movement or loosening of the teeth. There should not be any significant carries, gingivitis, periodontitis, or loose teeth. Although implants, caps, and crowns are not contraindications to an appliance, the caps and crowns should be assessed for stability because a loose cap or crown likely will be displaced when the appliance is removed (**Box 1**).

Severe bruxism is a relative contraindication because excess lateral motion during sleep may cause the appliance to come off the teeth and lead to damage to the appliance. Severe dental flattening caused by bruxism also affects the appliances retention. Ongoing TMJ pain is a contraindication because the appliance typically causes additional stress to the joint and worsens the pain. The patient should be examined to determine if there is any popping or crepitation in the TMJs with jaw opening, closing, or protrusion because TMJ irregularity may increase the risk of TMJ pain with appliance use. Examination also should assess how far the patient can protrude the mandible because approximately 6 mm may be required for an adequate response to a sleep oral appliance in many. Patients with an anterior open bite generally have limited jaw protrusion and are not good candidates for an appliance. Those with severe micrognathia may not be able to get the appliance into their mouth, and the impression trays may be too large to take impressions. Large tori may limit obtaining impressions, although single-use impression trays often can be ground down to allow shallow impressions. The patient should be questioned about potential future braces

---

Box 1
Contraindications for mandibular advancement devices

Loose teeth, significant dental carries, or periodontitis

Dental work, caps, crowns, implants, or braces planned in near future

Bruxism, if severe

TMJ crepitation, popping, or pain

Inadequate mandibular protrusion

Severe micrognathia

Large tori

Significant claustrophobia

Significant nasal obstruction

Large oropharyngeal masses or large tonsils

or dental work because significant changes to the dentition or bite require a remake of the appliance.

Some patients have severe enough claustrophobia that they may not be able to tolerate an appliance in their mouth with their mouth held closed. Nasal obstruction is a relative contraindication for a sleep oral appliance because increasing nasal resistance lowers the effectiveness of the appliance.[10] Even subjective nasal obstruction has been associated with reduced efficacy of a MAD in women.[11] In general, patients with severe nasal obstruction should have the cause of the obstruction treated with medication or surgery prior to beginning use of an appliance. In addition, the patient's upper airway anatomy has an impact on the effectiveness of a sleep oral appliance. Large tonsils and a very long palate and uvula likely reduce the effectiveness of an appliance.

The severity of a patient's sleep apnea should be assessed before considering an appliance. Historically, it was felt that cure rates were reduced in patients with severe sleep apnea, yet this was based on studies with small sample sizes. It is now recognized that there can be significant benefit from a sleep oral appliance regardless of the apnea severity and even a partial response to treatment is better than no treatment. In a long-term randomized controlled trial of MAD versus continuous positive airway pressure (CPAP) in mild to severe obstructive sleep apnea (OSA) patients, those treated with CPAP did better with reductions in apnea-hypopnea index (AHI) and oxyhemoglobin saturation but there was no statistical difference between the proportion of patients obtaining successful treatment. Successful treatment was obtained in 56% versus 60% in patients with nonsevere OSA and 50% versus 75% with severe OSA for MAD and CPAP, respectively, and there was no statistical difference in outcomes with the Epworth Sleepiness Scale (ESS), Functional Outcomes of Sleep Questionnaire (FOSQ), and SF-36-Item Short Form Health Survey. Other investigators studying patients with severe OSA found CPAP and MAD to have equal effectiveness in reducing the risk of fatal cardiovascular events.[12,13]

TYPES OF APPLIANCES

There are 3 types of sleep oral appliances: palatal lift appliances, TRDs, and mandibular advancement devices. Palatal lift appliances no longer are in clinical use whereas TRDs typically are used only if a mandibular advancement appliance cannot be used due to a lack of sufficient dentition. Mandibular advancement devices may be stock boil-and-bite appliances or customized devices. Custom devices may be either a single appliance attached to both mandible and maxilla with a fixed amount of protrusion (monobloc) or may be 2 separate pieces that are linked together, allowing adjustability and variable amounts of protrusion. There are hundreds of different designs that may be made from a variety of materials, including acrylic and nylon. Most appliances fit by physicians or dentist today are adjustable customized devices, which allow for creation of smaller devices, better dental retention, better lateral motion, and slow adjustment so as to reduce the risk of TMJ problems.

TRDs are stock items, available in different sizes, or may be custom made. There are not many studies on the efficacy of these devices, yet they appear to have similar efficacy to mandibular advancement appliances. TRDs have a lower compliance rate compared with MADs.[1,2]

FITTING PROCESS: IMPRESSIONS, BITE REGISTRATION, AND ADJUSTMENTS

Fitting a sleep oral appliance begins in the office by taking full upper and lower dental impressions. This can be done with a variety of materials, including alginate impression material mixed to correct timing and consistency or more durable impression material, such as hydrophilic vinyl poly siloxane. The impression material is placed into a properly sized impression tray and then compressed over the dentition and should include some of the gingivae so as to include the dental undercuts. Plaster cast stone models then are created from the impressions, either by the physician/dentist or by a dental laboratory. A bite registration is obtained, typically with a 5-mm vertical interincisor distance. A gauge is used to determine centric occlusion, maximum protrusion, maximum retrusion, and protrusal range (available from several vendors). The initial protrusion for the appliance is determined based on this information along with how much adjustability is possible with the planned appliance. The impressions and bite registration are sent to a dental laboratory for creation of stone models and the appliance. Digital imaging also can be used to obtain impressions, and some laboratories can create appliances made from biocompatible nylon materials directly from the digital images using 3-D printing. Initial positioning for a MAD typically is 50% of maximal protrusion.

EFFICACY OF ORAL APPLIANCE THERAPY

Treatment goals of any therapy should be to improve quality of life and life expectancy. Patients do not care if their AHI is lower or not unless they feel better, their bedpartners are happier, and they live healthier and longer. Nearly all research studies on sleep apnea treatments, however, focus on improving physiologic variables of sleep apnea because they are easier outcome measures than life expectancy. As a result, AHI, oxygen desaturation, and measures of sleep fragmentation have become the standards for measuring outcomes for most OSA treatments. Most studies use AHI reduced to less than 5 or 10 per hour or a reduction in AHI by more than 50% as the primary physiologic outcome measure and quality of life measured by a sleep questionnaire, such as the FOSQ or ESS.

Studies of custom mandibular advancement appliances have found a mean reduction of AHI from baseline in the range of 30% to 72%.[6,14–17] When looking at complete resolution of sleep apnea (treatment AHI <5/h) or partial resolution of sleep apnea (treatment AHI <50% of baseline AHI), success ranged from 45% to 100%.[6,14–17] Studies typically show a better success rate for patients with lower AHIs, because it is easier to achieve a final AHI less than 5 per hour when the starting AHI is lower. Other studies have shown benefits in arousal indices, amount of rapid eye movement (REM) sleep, oxygen saturation,[18–20] subjective snoring,[14,18–20] and subjective sleepiness.[14,18–20]

There also are several studies that have shown reduction in blood pressure in hypertensive patients with the use of oral appliance therapy,[21–23] although other studies have shown no benefit on blood pressure.[24]

MADs are effective in reducing AHI via a nonlinear dose-dependent relationship with degree of advancement, and greater protrusion often results in better outcomes.[25–30]

CPAP clearly is more effective than MADs in reducing AHI, as reported by multiple meta-analyses comparing the 2 therapies.[31–35] The most recent meta-analysis of 14 randomized controlled trials comparing efficacy of CPAP to oral appliances[35] found that compared with oral appliances, CPAP significantly decreased AHI, lowest oxygen saturation, and ESS but had no significant change in FOSQ or blood pressure. In contrast, oral appliances significantly improved REM percentage in the severe OSA groups and ESS in the adjustable oral appliance group. CPAP reduced AHI by an additional 8.43 events per hour over MAD, yet oral appliances were preferred to CPAP by patients.

Cardiovascular mortality was studied in 1 observational study of 570 subjects with severe OSA (AHI $\geq$30/h) and a control group of 269 subjects without sleep apnea (AHI <5/h), finding similar cardiovascular mortality with CPAP and with MAD. Those with OSA all were treated with CPAP and offered MAD if nonadherent with CPAP. With a follow-up of 79 months, cardiovascular mortality was studied in the 4 groups (no OSA, CPAP treatment, CPAP then MAD treatment, and those who declined treatment). The no-apnea group had the lowest cardiovascular mortality (0.28 per 100 person years), followed by the CPAP group (0.56 per 100 person years), and then the MAD group (0.61 per 100 person years), and the highest was in the untreated OSA group (2.1 per 100 person years).[36]

COMPLIANCE OF MANDIBULAR ADVANCEMENT APPLIANCES

Compliance with positive airway pressure (PAP) has been defined by Kribbs and colleagues[37] as using PAP for at least 4 hours a night for at least 5 nights a week (or a total of 20 hours a week), and this definition has been accepted by the American Academy of Sleep Medicine, Centers for Medicare & Medicaid Services, and essentially all third-party insurance payers in the United States. Because normal sleep time in a week is approximately 49 hours a week, the current definition of "compliant therapy" represents the use of PAP for 41% of normal sleep hours (20/49 = 41%). Published studies on PAP have shown that only 58% to 80% of patients accept PAP therapy,[38–40] and 49% of patients are compliant in the first month of therapy.[37] In one of the largest studies to date, the Apnea Positive Pressure Long-term Efficacy Study (APPLES) was a 6-month, randomized, double-blind, 2-arm, sham-controlled, multicenter trial on a total of 1516 enrolled subjects. In this study, when analyzing CPAP use over the prior month, the compliance rate at 6 months was only 39% in the active CPAP group.[41] Adherence to bilevel PAP and auto-adjusting PAP are the same as to CPAP. All PAP machines used in the United States now have built in compliance meters to allow a daily report of adherence to therapy.

There have been several publications on compliance with oral appliance therapy, although most report only on subjective compliance, with a range of continued use at 1 year from under 10% to as high as 76%.[11] In 1 study of 544 patients sent a questionnaire an average of 6 years after construction of the appliance, 251 patients returned the questionnaire and 161 continued use (64/%). The most common reasons to discontinue use were discomfort (44%) and no benefit (34%). Subjective MAD compliance was better than objective CPAP compliance by an average of 0.7 hours per night, according to the American Academy of Sleep Medicine task force,[31] and a meta-analysis of 6 studies using both subjective and objective measures found compliance with MAD to be 1.1 hours a night more than CPAP.[34] Objective measures of compliance with MAD after 3 months of treatment found a mean use of 6.4 hours to 6.6 hours a night.[42,43] Oral appliances typically are preferred to CPAP in most crossover studies comparing the 2 modes of therapy.[31,44] Despite a lower efficacy of MAD versus CPAP, it is likely that better compliance/adherence with therapy allows MADs to improve overall effectiveness. Unfortunately, most oral appliances in use today do not have any way to measure objective adherence with therapy, so objective compliance in an individual patient is not possible.

AVOIDANCE AND TREATMENT OF COMPLICATIONS OF MANDIBULAR ADVANCEMENT DEVICES

Complications/side effects frequently are associated with use of a sleep oral appliance, as listed in **Box 2**. Patients should be advised of the more common side effects

---

Box 2
Complications and side effects from oral appliances

TMJ side effects
  Transient or persistent TMJ pain
  Tenderness of muscles of mastication
  TMJ popping or crepitation
  Mouth or dental pain

Damage to dentition or dental restorations
  Tooth mobility
  Tooth fractures
  Damage to crowns, caps, implants, or retainers

Soft tissue–related complications
  Tongue ulcerations/sores/irritation
  Drooling
  Dry mouth
  Gingival irritation and ulceration

Occlusal changes
  Decreased overjet and overbite
  Movement of mandibular molars and premolars
  Altered occlusal contacts and bite changes
  Interproximal gaps
  Angulation of incisors

Appliance-related complications
  Inadequate retention on the teeth/falling off during use
  Appliance breakage
  Excess gagging
  Anxiety/claustrophobia issues

---

and asked to come in for any significant problems because early intervention may help resolve a problem before it worsens.

Drooling and increased salivation are common in the first week or 2 of use, in up to 60% of patients,[45] but typically subside as patients increase use. Use of a towel over a pillow for the first week often prevents staining of their sheets and pillow cases. Ulceration and sores on the tongue may occur in up to 8% of patients[46] if there is insufficient room for the tongue in the mouth or the patient protrudes the tongue against a part of the appliance. As the mandible is slowly protruded, the problem typically resolves as more room is created for the tongue. On occasion, a different appliance design may be needed. Dry mouth also is common as a long-term issue, occurring up to 86% of patients,[47] although patients rarely are bothered by it.

Pain in 1 tooth or several teeth, occurring in up to 59% of patients,[47] usually means there is excess pressure from the appliance on those teeth. The appliance should be trimmed or ground down in that area, to eliminate the pressure on the affected teeth. If not treated early, the tooth will likely loosen or move. For loose teeth, it is important to inspect the appliance for any pressure on the loose tooth and trim the appliance as needed to eliminate the excess dental pressure. If persisting, use of the appliance may need to be discontinued. If a cap or crown becomes loose or comes off, it is simple for a patient's dentist to cement it back on as long as the underlying tooth is healthy.

Abnormal occlusion on awakening is common, because the appliance protrudes the mandible during sleep, and on awakening, the mandible does not shift back to its normal position. Patients perceive that their bite is abnormal on awakening and they may be unable to chew or bite food normally or may have mild discomfort in the TMJ. If the mandible does not shift back there may be a permanent change in bite/occlusion and patients slowly shift to class III malocclusion. This problem typically is prevented by having a patient wear a morning aligner for 10 minutes to 30 minutes each morning, which repositions the mandible back to the normal bite each morning. The morning aligner is made by having the patient bite into a thermo-occlusal material, when first fitting the appliance, so as to capture the patient's normal bite. The patient then wears the aligner every morning, squeezing the teeth together for 10 seconds and then relaxing for a minute, and repeats the process for at least 10 minutes, or until the bite is back to normal.

TMJ pain and dysfunction are common in patients with underlying TMJ problems but also may occur in patients without TMJ issues or from just from wearing the appliance or may be due to too rapid or excessive protrusion of the appliance. Overall, TMJ pain occurs in up to 37% of patients.[48] Typical instructions are to protrude the appliance slowly, 0.5mm twice a week, and to discontinue protrusion and instead retrude a few millimeters if experiencing any TMJ pain. If any TMJ pain occurs, patients can be treated with nonsteroidal anti-inflammatory agents, warm compresses, and either retruding the appliance or discontinuing use until the pain subsides. When resuming use, the appliance should be retruded, so there is less stress on the TMJ.

Shifting of the teeth should be an uncommon event because the appliance acts as a retainer, that is, it retains the same position of the teeth relative to one another because the appliance does not change shape. As long as it is worn nightly, the appliance should maintain dental position. Boil-and-bite appliances, however, often cause excessive pressure on the incisors, leading to angulation of incisors, a decreased overjet and overbite, and altered occlusal contacts and bite changes. Even custom appliances can become distorted by wear and tear or severe bruxism. If the appliance changes shape, then it leads to problems with retention and dental motion over time. Regular office checks are important to avoid these problems. A bigger issue is a change in the bite caused by a change in the TMJ, with occlusion becoming more class III over time. The problem is more frequent if patients do not use their morning aligner. Once a change in bite occurs, it is difficult to treat. Some patients prefer the new jaw position, although others find it causes difficulty biting foods and chewing. Treatment options include discontinuation of the appliance, manually putting posterior pressure on the mentum several times a day, use of orthodontics, and mandibular retrusion surgery. Temporary morning occlusal changes or long-term occlusal changes occur in up to 41% of patients.[49] Prevention is the best approach, by using the morning aligner regularly and checking patient progress every 3 months to 6 months.

DISCLOSURE

The author has nothing to disclose.

REFERENCES

1. Sutherland K, Deane SA, Chan AS, et al. Comparative effects of two oral appliances on upper airway structure in obstructive sleep apnea. Sleep 2011;34(4):469–77.
2. Deane SA, Cistulli PA, Ng AT, et al. Comparison of mandibular advancement splint and tongue stabilizing device in obstructive sleep apnea: a randomized controlled trial. Sleep 2009;32(5):648–53.
3. Chan AS, Sutherland K, Schwab RJ, et al. The effect of mandibular advancement on upper airway structure in obstructive sleep apnoea. Thorax 2010;65:726–32.

4. Ryan CF, Love LL, Peat D, et al. Mandibular advancement oral appliance therapy for obstructive sleep apnoea: effect on awake calibre of the velopharynx. Thorax 1999;54:972–7.

5. Brown EC, Cheng S, McKenzie DK, et al. Respiratory movement of upper airway tissue in obstructive sleep apnea. Sleep 2013;36:1069–76.

6. Petri N, Svanholt P, Solow B, et al. Mandibular advancement appliance for obstructive sleep apnoea: results of a randomised placebo controlled trial using parallel group design. J Sleep Res 2008;17:221–9.

7. de Almeida FR, Bittencourt LR, de Almeida CI, et al. Effects of mandibular posture on obstructive sleep apnea severity and the temporomandibular joint in patients fitted with an oral appliance. Sleep 2002;25:507–13.

8. Kato J, Isono S, Tanaka A, et al. Dose-dependent effects of mandibular advancement on pharyngeal mechanics and nocturnal oxygenation in patients with sleep-disordered breathing. Chest 2000;117:1065–72.

9. Kuna ST, Woodson LC, Solanki DR, et al. Effect of progressive mandibular advancement on pharyngeal airway size in anesthetized adults. Anesthesiology 2008;109:605–12.

10. Zeng B, Ng AT, Qian J, et al. Influence of nasal resistance on oral appliance treatment outcome in obstructive sleep apnea. Sleep 2008;31(4):543–7.

11. Marklund M, Stenlund H, Franklin KA. Mandibular advancement devices in 630 men and women with obstructive sleep apnea and snoring. Chest 2004;125:1270–8.

12. Almeida FR, Bansback N. Long-term effectiveness of oral appliance versus CPAP therapy and the emerging importance of understanding patient preferences. Sleep 2013;36(9):1271–2.

13. Doff MHJ, Hoekema A, Wijkstra PJ, et al. Oral appliance versus continuous positive airway pressure in obstructive sleep apnea syndrome: a 2-year follow-up. Sleep 2013;36:1289–96.

14. Blanco J, Zamarron C, Abeleira Pazos MT, et al. Prospective evaluation of an oral appliance in the treatment of obstructive sleep apnea syndrome. Sleep Breath 2005;9:20–5.

15. Vanderveken OM, Devolder A, Marklund M, et al. Comparison of a custom-made and a thermoplastic oral appliance for the treatment of mild sleep apnea. Am J Respir Crit Care Med 2008;178:197–202.

16. Quinnell TG, Bennett M, Jordan J, et al. A crossover randomised controlled trial of oral mandibular advancement devices for obstructive sleep apnoeahypopnoea (TOMADO). Thorax 2014;69:938–45.

17. Aarab G, Lobbezoo F, Heymans MW, et al. Longterm follow-up of a randomized controlled trial of oral appliance therapy in obstructive sleep apnea. Respiration 2011;82:162–8.

18. Gotsopoulos H, Chen C, Qian J, et al. Oral appliance therapy improves symptoms in obstructive sleep apnea: A randomized, controlled trial. Am J Respir Crit Care Med 2002;166:743–8.

19. Johnston CD, Gleadhill IC, Cinnamond MJ, et al. Mandibular advancement appliances and obstructive sleep apnoea: a randomized clinical trial. Eur J Orthod 2002;24:251–62.

20. Mehta A, Qian J, Petocz P, et al. A randomized, controlled study of a mandibular advancement splint for obstructive sleep apnea. Am J Respir Crit Care Med 2001;163:1457–61.

21. Andrén A, Hedberg P, Walker-Engstrom ML, et al. Effects of treatment with oral appliance on 24-h blood pressure in patients with obstructive sleep apnea and hypertension: a randomized clinical trial. Sleep Breath 2013;17:705–12.

22. Gotsopoulos H, Kelly JJ, Cistulli PA. Oral appliance therapy reduces blood pressure in obstructive sleep apnea: a randomized, controlled trial. Sleep 2004;27: 934–41.

23. Bratton DJ, Gaisl T, Wons AM, et al. CPAP vs mandibular advancement devices and blood pressure in patients with obstructive sleep apnea: a systematic review and meta-analysis. JAMA 2015;314:2280–93.

24. Phillips CL, Grunstein RR, Darendeliler MA, et al. Health outcomes of continuous positive airway pressure versus oral appliance treatment for obstructive sleep apnea: a randomized controlled trial. Am J Respir Crit Care Med 2013;187:879–87.

25. Raphaelson MA, Alpher EJ, Bakker KW, et al. Oral appliance therapy for obstructive sleep apnea syndrome: progressive mandibular advancement during polysomnography. Cranio 1998;16(1):44–50.

26. Tsai WH, Vazquez JC, Oshima T, et al. Remotely controlled mandibular positioner predicts efficacy of oral appliances in sleep apnea. Am J Respir Crit Care Med 2004;170(4):366–70.

27. Gindre L, Gagnadoux F, Meslier N, et al. Mandibular advancement for obstructive sleep apnea: dose effect on apnea, long-term use and tolerance. Respiration 2008;76(4):386–92.

28. Almeida FR, Parker JA, Hodges JS, et al. Effect of a titration polysomnogram on treatment success with a mandibular repositioning appliance. J Clin Sleep Med 2009;5(3):198–204.

29. Aarab G, Lobbezoo F, Hamburger HL, et al. Effects of an oral appliance with different mandibular protrusion positions at a constant vertical dimension on obstructive sleep apnea. Clin Oral Investig 2010;14(3):339–45.

30. Dort L, Remmers J. A combination appliance for obstructive sleep apnea: the effectiveness of mandibular advancement and tongue retention. J Clin Sleep Med 2012;8(3):265–9.

31. Ramar K, Dort LC, Katz SG, et al. Clinical practice guideline for the treatment of obstructive sleep apnea and snoring with oral appliance therapy: an update for 2015. An American Academy of Sleep Medicine and American Academy of Dental Sleep Medicine Clinical Practice Guideline. J Clin Sleep Med 2015; 11(7):773–827.

32. Giles TL, Lasserson TJ, Smith BH, et al. Continuous positive airways pressure for obstructive sleep apnoea in adults. Cochrane Database Syst Rev 2006;(3):CD001106.

33. Lim J, Lasserson TJ, Fleetham J, et al. Oral appliances for obstructive sleep apnoea. Cochrane Database Syst Rev 2006;(1):CD004435.

34. Schwartz M, Acosta L, Hung YL, et al. Effects of CPAP and mandibular advancement device Oral Appliances in Management of OSA treatment in obstructive sleep apnea patients: a systematic review and meta-analysis. Sleep Breath 2018;22(3):555–68.

35. Zhang M, Liu Y, Liu Y, et al. Effectiveness of oral appliances versus continuous positive airway pressure in treatment of OSA patients: an updated meta-analysis. Cranio 2018;37(6):347–64.

36. Anandam A, Patil M, Akinnusi M, et al. Cardiovascular mortality in obstructive sleep apnoea treated with continuous positive airway pressure or oral appliance: an observational study. Respirology 2013;18(8):1184–90.

37. Kribbs NB, Pack AI, Kline LR, et al. Objective measurement of patterns of nasal CPAP use by patients with obstructive sleep apnea. Am Rev Respir Dis 1993; 147(4):887–95.
38. Waldhorn RE, Herrick TW, Nguyen MC, et al. Long-term compliance with nasal continuous positive airway pressure therapy of obstructive sleep apnea. Chest 1990;97:33–8.
39. Meurice JC, Dore P, Paquereau J, et al. Predictive factors of long term compliance with nasal continuous positive airway pressure treatment in sleep apnea syndrome. Chest 1994;105:429–33.
40. Rauscher H, Formanek D, Popp W, et al. Nasal CPAP and weight loss in hypertensive patients with obstructive sleep apnea. Thorax 1993;48:529–33.
41. Kushida CA, Nichols DA, Holmes TH, et al. Effects of continuous positive airway pressure on neurocognitive function in obstructive sleep apnea patients: The Apnea Positive Pressure Long-term Efficacy Study (APPLES). Sleep 2012;35(12): 1593–602.
42. Dieltjens M, Verbruggen AE, Braem MJ, et al. Determinants of objective compliance during oral appliance therapy in patients with sleep-disordered breathing: a prospective clinical trial. JAMA Otolaryngol Head Neck Surg 2015;141(10): 894–900.
43. Vanderveken OM, Dieltjens M, Wouters K, et al. Objective measurement of compliance during oral appliance therapy for sleep-disordered breathing. Thorax 2013;68(1):91–6.
44. Sutherland K, Phillips CL, Cistulli PA. Efficacy versus effectiveness in the treatment of obstructive sleep apnea: CPAP and oral appliances. J Dent Sleep Med 2015;2(4):175–81.
45. Dort LC, Hussein J. Snoring and obstructive sleep apnea: compliance with oral appliance therapy. J Otolaryngol 2004;33:172–6.
46. de Almeida FR, Lowe AA, Tsuiki S, et al. Long term compliance and side effects of oral appliances used for the treatment of snoring and obstructive sleep apnea syndrome. J Clin Sleep Med 2005;1:143–52.
47. Fritsch KM, Iseli A, Russi EW, et al. Side effects of mandibular advancement devices for sleep apnea treatment. Am J Respir Crit Care Med 2001;164:813–8.
48. McGown AD, Makker HK, Battagel JM, et al. Long-term use of mandibular advancement splints for snoring and obstructive sleep apnea: a quesionnaire survey. Eur Respir J 2001;17:462–6.
49. Marklund M, Sahlin C, Stenlund H, et al. Mandibular advancement device in patients with obstructive apnea: long-term effects on apnea and sleep. Chest 2001; 120:162–9.

Surgical and Nonsurgical Weight Loss for Patients with Obstructive Sleep Apnea

Katherine H. Saunders, MD, DABOM*, Leon I. Igel, MD, FTOS, DABOM,
Beverly G. Tchang, MD, DABOM

KEYWORDS

- Overweight • Obesity • Weight management • Pharmacotherapy
- Antiobesity medications • Bariatric surgery • Devices • Sleep apnea

KEY POINTS

- Weight loss can improve apnea-hypopnea index and is an essential part of the treatment plan for patients with obstructive sleep apnea and overweight or obesity.
- Lifestyle interventions including diet, physical activity, and behavioral modifications are the cornerstones of weight management.
- Many patients require advanced therapies, such as antiobesity medications, bariatric surgery, and/or devices, to achieve and maintain clinically significant weight loss.
- Successful treatment of overweight and obesity requires a multidisciplinary approach to counteract the body's resistance to weight loss.
- Health care providers who treat patients with sleep apnea should be familiar with the medical and surgical options available to patients with overweight and obesity.

INTRODUCTION

The relationship between obesity and obstructive sleep apnea (OSA) is complex. Many epidemiologic studies have revealed a strong association between excess weight and OSA in that most individuals with moderate to severe OSA also have an elevated body mass index (BMI).[1] Early hypotheses for a causative relationship between OSA and obesity proposed a cycle in which OSA led to metabolic dysfunction and obesity led to OSA. Animal models have provided potential mechanisms for this relationship. The pathophysiology of OSA involves chronic intermittent hypoxia resulting in systemic and organ-specific inflammation, which cascades into adipocyte dysfunction, gut microbiota dysbiosis, and eventual weight gain.[2] The pathophysiology of obesity can involve excess pharyngeal adipose tissue, which leads to airway

Division of Endocrinology, Diabetes and Metabolism, Comprehensive Weight Control Center, Weill Cornell Medicine, 1165 York Avenue, New York, NY 10065, USA
* Corresponding author.
E-mail address: kph2001@med.cornell.edu

Otolaryngol Clin N Am 53 (2020) 409–420
https://doi.org/10.1016/j.otc.2020.02.003
0030-6665/20/© 2020 Elsevier Inc. All rights reserved.

narrowing, and excess abdominal and chest wall fat, which reduces lung volumes, thus contributing to sleep-disordered breathing.[3]

Weight loss has long been considered a therapeutic intervention for the treatment of OSA because of the possible causative relationship between obesity and OSA. The Wisconsin Sleep Disorder study, a longitudinal prospective cohort study, found that weight loss of about 10% predicted a 26% reduction in the apnea-hypopnea index (AHI).[4] Subsequent randomized-controlled trials (RCTs) consistently demonstrated an improvement in AHI with significant weight loss.[5] Three trials, one RCT[6] and two prospective observational extensions of RCTs,[7,8] provided 1-year data showing a greater chance of OSA remission with greater weight loss and weight loss mainte-nance. In the Sleep AHEAD trial, participants with type 2 diabetes, obesity, and severe OSA were randomized to intensive lifestyle intervention or standard diabetes educa-tion.[6] Mean weight loss was 10.8 kg in the intensive lifestyle intervention group versus 0.6 kg in the control group, and 13.6% of the intensive lifestyle intervention group achieved OSA remission at 1 year, compared with 3.5% of the control group.

The direct relationship between weight loss and OSA improvement is further sup-ported by the bariatric literature. In a meta-analysis of RCTs, nonrandomized controlled trials, and uncontrolled case series, Roux-en-Y gastric bypass (RYGB) sur-gery was associated with a reduction in the number of apneas or hypopneas by 33.85 events per hour.[9] Mean weight loss in this surgical cohort was 43.5 kg, and 86.6% re-ported resolution of OSA. Because trends in bariatric surgery have seen less laparo-scopic adjustable gastric banding (LAGB) and more laparoscopic sleeve gastrectomy (LSG) over the past 20 years, a systematic review and meta-analysis is planned to assess these newer procedures and associated outcomes.[10]

The effect of OSA treatment, specifically continuous positive airway pressure, on obesity has been heterogeneous until a recent meta-analysis was performed to address this question. Drager and colleagues[11] conducted a meta-analysis of 29 RCTs and concluded that continuous positive airway pressure initiation and use in in-dividuals with overweight and obesity was associated with a statistically significant greater weight gain of about 0.5 kg compared with control subjects. The mechanism for weight gain is unclear but may involve a reduction in basal metabolic rate without a corresponding reduction in energy intake, in addition to subtle changes in dietary and eating behaviors.[12] Furthermore, the addition of continuous positive airway pressure to weight loss in the management of OSA has not been shown to be superior to weight loss alone in regards to some metabolic endpoints.[13] As a result, weight management has become an increasingly integral part of the OSA treatment plan among patients with overweight and obesity.

Successful treatment of overweight and obesity requires a multidisciplinary approach to counteract the body's resistance to weight loss. Although diet, physical activity, and behavioral modifications are the cornerstones of weight management, many patients require additional interventions, such as antiobesity medications and/ or bariatric surgery, to achieve and maintain clinically significant weight loss. In this article, we review the available treatment strategies for overweight and obesity including lifestyle modifications, medications and devices approved by the US Food and Drug Administration (FDA), and bariatric surgery.

LIFESTYLE MODIFICATIONS AND DRUG-INDUCED WEIGHT GAIN

Many dietary strategies are effective for weight loss, and there are no data illustrating one best approach. Because adherence to diet is associated with increased weight loss, recommendations should be customized to a patient's preferences.[14] Patients should be counseled to limit sugary drinks, junk food, and sweets, because diets rich in ultraprocessed food can lead to excess calorie intake and weight gain.[15] Many patients with OSA also have insulin resistance so a low-glycemic-index diet is a good option to curb hunger and decrease cravings by reducing blood sugar fluctuations.[16] A Mediterranean diet has been shown to reduce the incidence of major cardiovascular events and is a reasonable option for patients with OSA because they are generally at high cardiovascular risk.[17,18] Registered dietitians can provide dietary education and customize diet plans.

The American College of Sports Medicine recommends 150 minutes of moderate-intensity aerobic physical activity (eg, brisk walking), 75 minutes of vigorous-intensity aerobic physical activity (eg, jogging), or an equivalent combination per week.[19] Resistance training or muscle strengthening is also recommended at least twice weekly. Because some patients with OSA have comorbidities limiting their mobility, they should be encouraged to perform tolerable exercise even if they cannot meet the previously mentioned recommendations. Exercise physiologists and physical therapists can provide support for patients.

Behavioral interventions for weight loss include self-monitoring, such as tracking food intake or recording weights. Stress reduction can also be helpful for weight loss. An interdisciplinary team including physicians, dietitians, sports physiologists, physical therapists, psychologists, social workers, and other health care professionals can provide customized support for patients. Because weight maintenance is often much more difficult than initial weight loss, it is important that patients continue regular follow-up with their providers to ensure long-term adherence to their individualized care plans.

Multiple medications are associated with weight gain, including certain antidiabetic, antihypertensive, antidepressant, antipsychotic, antiepileptic, and antihistamine agents, and steroids, contraceptives, and other hormonal agents.[20] Patients with OSA are frequently on medications that can lead to significant weight gain, such as sleep aides diphenhydramine, trazodone, amitriptyline, nortriptyline, and mirtazapine. Patients' medication lists should be reviewed carefully, and the benefits of treatment should be balanced against the probability of weight gain.[21] When possible, providers should recommend weight-neutral or weight loss–promoting medications. If there are no alternative medications, weight gain is prevented or reduced by selecting the lowest dose/frequency required for clinical efficacy for the shortest duration necessary.

ANTIOBESITY MEDICATIONS

Weight loss achieved by lifestyle modifications alone is often limited and difficult to maintain because of adaptive physiologic responses and alterations in hormones, which lead to an increase in appetite and a reduction in metabolic rate.[22–25] Antiobesity pharmacotherapy (**Table 1**) can offset changes in appetite and energy expenditure and improve adherence to lifestyle interventions. Antiobesity pharmacotherapy is considered in patients with OSA who have a BMI greater than or equal to 27 kg/m^2.[26,27]

Many of the medications signal through noradrenergic or dopaminergic pathways and target the arcuate nucleus of the hypothalamus to stimulate the anorexigenic pro-opiomelanocortin neurons. Because obesity is a chronic, relapsing disease, medications should be used long-term as an adjunct to diet and exercise. The five main antiobesity medications approved by the FDA are (1) phentermine, (2) orlistat, (3) phentermine/topiramate extended-release (ER), (4) naltrexone sustained-release

Table 1
Most commonly prescribed antiobesity medications approved by the FDA

Medication	Mechanism, Dosage, Formulation	Total Body Weight Loss (%)[a]	FDA Approval	Schedule IV Controlled Substance
Phentermine (Adipex,[33] Lomaira[34])	Adrenergic agonist 8–37.5 mg daily (8-mg dose can be prescribed up to TID) Capsule, tablet	15 mg/d: 6.1 7.5 mg/d: 5.5 Placebo: 1.7 28 wk[32]	1959	Yes
Phentermine/ topiramate extended-release (Qsymia[37])	Adrenergic agonist/ neurostabilizer 3.75/23–15/92 mg daily Capsule	15/92 mg/d: 9.8 7.5/46 mg daily: 7.8 Placebo: 1.2 56 wk[36]	2012	Yes
Naltrexone sustained-release/ bupropion sustained-release (Contrave[41])	Opioid receptor antagonist/dopamine and norepinephrine reuptake inhibitor 8/90 mg daily to 16/180 mg BID Tablet	16/180 mg BID: 6.1 8/180 mg BID: 5.0 Placebo: 1.3 56 wk[40]	2014	No
Liraglutide 3.0 mg (Saxenda[43])	GLP-1 receptor agonist 0.6–3.0 mg daily Prefilled pen, subcutaneous injection	3.0 mg daily: 8.0 Placebo: 2.6 56 wk[42]	2014	No
Orlistat (Alli,[47] Xenical[46])	Lipase inhibitor 60–120 mg TID with meals Capsule	120 mg TID: 9.6 Placebo: 5.6 52 wk[45]	1999	No

Abbreviations: BID, twice daily; GLP-1, glucagon-like peptide-1; TID, three times daily.
 [a] Intention-to-treat analyses.

(SR)/bupropion SR, and (5) liraglutide 3.0 mg.[28–30] In addition to promoting weight loss, each medication can improve a variety of comorbidities common to patients with OSA including type 2 diabetes, hypertension, and hyperlipidemia.

Phentermine

Phentermine, approved by the FDA in 1959, is the most commonly prescribed antiobesity medication in the United States.[31] It is an adrenergic agonist indicated for short-term use because there are no long-term safety trials of phentermine monotherapy. However, it was approved in combination with topiramate ER for long-term treatment so many providers prescribe phentermine monotherapy off-label for longer durations. In a 28-week RCT, participants assigned to phentermine, 15 mg daily, lost an average of 6.0 kg compared with 1.5 kg among the group assigned to lifestyle intervention alone.[32] Dosage should be individualized to achieve response with the lowest effective dose.[33,34] Phentermine is a schedule IV controlled substance. The most common treatment-emergent adverse events (TEAEs) include increased heart rate, headache, insomnia, and dry mouth. Contraindications include pregnancy, cardiovascular disease, hyperthyroidism, and glaucoma. Because some patients with OSA have cardiovascular disease, other antiobesity agents might be more appropriate for this population; however, phentermine might be useful to address residual daytime sleepiness related to OSA (treated or untreated) if there are no contraindications for use, such as evidence of cardiovascular disease.

Phentermine/Topiramate Extended-Release

There are many mechanisms and hormonal pathways responsible for appetite regulation. Targeting different appetite-regulating pathways simultaneously with combinations of low-dose medications can have an additive or synergistic effect on weight loss while reducing the risk of TEAEs often experienced on higher doses of individual therapies. Phentermine/topiramate extended-release, approved in 2012, combines low doses of phentermine and topiramate, the latter of which was initially approved for epilepsy and migraine prophylaxis. Topiramate reduces caloric intake by inhibiting carbonic anhydrase, antagonizing glutamate, and modulating γ-aminobutyric acid receptors.[35] In a randomized, double-blind, placebo-controlled trial, participants on phentermine/topiramate ER 15/92 mg lost 9.8 kg compared with 7.8 kg among those assigned to 7.5/46 mg and 1.2 kg among those assigned to lifestyle modifications alone after 56 weeks.[36] Phentermine/topiramate ER is a schedule IV controlled substance available in four doses (3.75/23 mg, 7.5/46 mg, 11.25/69 mg, 15.0/92 mg), which should be prescribed according to a dose-escalation protocol.[37] The FDA requires a Risk Evaluation and Mitigation Strategy to reduce the risk of orofacial clefts in infants exposed during pregnancy.[38] The most common TEAEs include increased heart rate, headache, paresthesia, and insomnia. Contraindications include pregnancy, cardiovascular disease, hyperthyroidism, and glaucoma. Although this combination medication allows lower doses of each component, caution should be used when prescribing to patients with OSA because they are often at higher cardiovascular risk. Similar to phentermine, in appropriately selected populations, phentermine/topiramate ER might be a useful option to address residual daytime sleepiness related to OSA (treated or untreated) if there are no contraindications for use, such as evidence of cardiovascular disease.

Naltrexone Sustained-Release/Bupropion Sustained-Release

Bupropion is a dopamine and norepinephrine reuptake inhibitor, which is approved as an antidepressant and as an aide for smoking cessation. Naltrexone, an opioid antagonist, is approved to treat opioid dependence and alcohol abuse. The combination was approved in 2014 and reduces appetite and food cravings by targeting the arcuate nucleus of the hypothalamus and the mesolimbic dopamine reward circuit.[39] In a randomized, double-blind, placebo-controlled trial, mean change in weight was 6.1% in the group assigned naltrexone 32 mg/bupropion 360 mg daily compared with 5.0% in the group assigned naltrexone 16 mg/bupropion 360 mg daily and 1.3% in the group assigned to lifestyle intervention alone after 56 weeks.[40] Each tablet contains 8 mg of naltrexone SR and 90 mg of bupropion SR, which should be prescribed according to a dose-escalation protocol.[41] The most common TEAEs include headache, nausea, vomiting, and constipation. Naltrexone/bupropion is contraindicated in pregnant patients and those taking chronic opioids and patients with uncontrolled hypertension, history of seizures, or conditions that predispose to seizure. Although there has been no completed cardiovascular outcome trial examining naltrexone/bupropion, it seems to be a reasonable option in patients with OSA who may be at higher cardiovascular risk if their blood pressure is well-controlled.

Liraglutide 3.0 mg

Liraglutide 3.0 mg is a glucagon-like peptide-1 receptor agonist approved in 2014 for the treatment of obesity that was initially approved at a lower dose (1.8 mg) for the treatment of type 2 diabetes. Mechanistically, it delays gastric emptying leading to reduced hunger and food intake. In a 56-week, randomized, placebo-controlled, double-blind trial, mean weight loss was 8.0% with liraglutide 3.0 mg daily, 4.7% with 1.8 mg daily, and 2.6% with lifestyle intervention alone.[42] Liraglutide is administered as a subcutaneous injection once daily according to a dose-escalation protocol.[43] The most common TEAEs include nausea, vomiting, diarrhea, and constipation. Liraglutide is contraindicated in pregnant patients and patients with personal or family history of medullary thyroid carcinoma or multiple endocrine neoplasia syndrome type 2. Thyroid C-cell tumors were found in rodents administered supratherapeutic doses of liraglutide, but there have been no published case reports of liraglutide leading to C-cell tumors in humans. The 1.8-mg dosage of liraglutide has been approved for cardiovascular risk reduction among patients with type 2 diabetes at elevated cardiovascular risk.[44] As a result, the higher dose of liraglutide might be an attractive option for patients with OSA who have cardiovascular risk factors.

Orlistat

Orlistat, which was approved in 1999, promotes weight loss by inhibiting lipase, thereby reducing dietary fat absorption. In a double-blind, randomized trial, mean weight loss was 9.6% among those assigned to orlistat, 120 mg three times per day, compared with 5.6% among those assigned to lifestyle interventions alone after 1 year.[45] The recommended dosage of orlistat is 120 mg (prescription-strength) or 60 mg (over-the-counter) three times a day.[46,47] Orlistat is not commonly prescribed for weight loss because of the TEAEs of steatorrhea, fecal urgency, fecal incontinence, and abdominal discomfort. Orlistat should not be used in patients who are pregnant or those who have cholestasis or chronic malabsorption syndromes.

BARIATRIC SURGERY

Bariatric surgery (**Table 2**) is the most effective treatment of obesity and, as a result, can lead to the greatest reduction in the AHI among patients with OSA. The three most common bariatric procedures in the United States are LSG, RYGB, and LAGB.[48] Bariatric surgery is considered in patients with OSA who have a BMI greater than or equal to 35 kg/m^2 and are motivated to lose weight, but have not achieved sufficient weight loss for target health goals following behavioral treatment, with or without pharmacotherapy.[26,49] Long-term medical follow-up and lifestyle changes are crucial for significant and sustained weight loss; however, most patients regain a portion of the lost weight. LSG and RYGB are performed more frequently than LAGB because of greater efficacy and tolerability. Contraindications include poor cardiac reserve, respiratory dysfunction, severe psychological disorders, and poor adherence to medical treatment.[50]

Laparoscopic Sleeve Gastrectomy

LSG removes approximately 70% of the stomach along the greater curvature. The fundus, which secretes the hunger hormone, ghrelin, is removed. The remaining stomach is shaped like a tube or a sleeve, and the pyloric valve remains intact. LSG is associated with 25% total body weight loss (TBWL) at 1 year.[51] There is a lower risk of nutritional deficiencies with LSG compared with RYGB because LSG is restrictive compared with RYGB, which is restrictive and malabsorptive. Sleeve gastrectomy is generally associated with fewer complications than RYGB and LAGB. Early adverse events include leakage along the staple line, bleeding, stenosis, gastroesophageal reflux, and vomiting; late complications include stomach expansion, leading to decreased restriction.[50] Unlike the other two procedures, LSG is not reversible.

Roux-en-Y Gastric Bypass

The RYGB attaches a small pouch created from the proximal stomach to the jejunum, thereby bypassing the remainder of the stomach, duodenum, and most of the jejunum. The procedure is associated with 30% TBWL at 1 year and greater improvements in weight-related health outcomes and mortality compared with LSG and LAGB.[51] There is a lower rate of gastroesophageal reflux following RYGB compared with LSG, and RYGB can even improve symptoms of reflux. Early adverse events include obstruction, stricture, leak, and failure of the staple line; late adverse events include nutritional deficiencies and anastomosis ulceration.[50] Dumping syndrome can develop at any time. The RYGB is reversible; however, it is generally only reversed under extreme circumstances.

Laparoscopic Adjustable Gastric Band

LAGB is an inflatable band placed around the fundus of the stomach to produce a small, proximal pouch. The size of the pouch is adjusted by adding or removing saline through a subcutaneous access port. The LAGB is associated with 15% to 20% TBWL at 1 year.[51,52] The procedure is less invasive than LSG and RYGB, but it is associated with more complications. The most common adverse events include nausea/vomiting, obstruction, band erosion/migration, and esophageal dysmotility leading to reflux.[53]

Table 2
Most commonly performed bariatric surgeries

Procedure	Description	Total Body Weight Loss at 1 Year (%)	Serious Perioperative Adverse Events (%)	Reversibility	Procedures Performed in 2013 (%)
LSG	~70% of stomach removed along greater curvature	25	1	No	43
RYGB	Small pouch (~<50 mL) is created from proximal stomach and attached to the jejunum; bypasses 95% of stomach, duodenum, and most of jejunum	30	5	Yes (but rarely done)	49
LAGB	Inflatable silicone band placed around fundus of stomach to create small pouch (~30 mL); pouch size is adjusted by increasing or decreasing quantity of saline in band via subcutaneous access port	15–20	5	Yes	6

Data from Heymsfield SB, Wadden TA. Mechanisms, pathophysiology, and management of obesity. N Engl J Med. 2017;376:254–6.

The LAGB is reversible and, in fact, many bands are eventually removed because of insufficient weight loss and/or adverse events.

ANTIOBESITY DEVICES

Devices to treat obesity (**Table 3**) are emerging options for patients with OSA who have contraindications to surgery and cannot achieve clinically meaningful weight loss with antiobesity pharmacotherapy.[54] The available options are reversible and minimally invasive. In addition, some are potentially more effective than antiobesity medications and safer for poor surgical candidates. The five FDA-approved devices include two intragastric balloons (Orbera [Apollo Endosurgery, Austin, TX] and Obalon [Obalon Theraputics Inc., Carlsbad, CA]), the AspireAssist aspiration device (Aspire Bariatrics, King of Prussia, PA), superabsorbent hydrogel capsules (Plenity, Gelesis, Boston, MA), and the TransPyloric Shuttle device (BAROnova Inc., San Carlos, CA). Although the devices are not currently widely used, they might be attractive options for patients with sleep apnea in the future.

Intragastric Balloons

The Orbera Intragastric Balloon System was approved in 2015 and the Obalon Balloon System was approved in 2016 for patients with a BMI of 30 to 40 kg/m^2.[55,56] Intragastric balloons are space-occupying devices, which are placed in the stomach to reduce functional gastric volume. Orbera is positioned endoscopically and filled with 400 to 700 mL of saline. It is then removed endoscopically after 6 months. In comparison, the Obalon system is comprised of three balloons that are swallowed as capsules and each filled with 250 mL of gas. They are placed sequentially over 3 months. Six months after the first balloon is placed, the balloons are removed endoscopically. TBWL ranges from 6.6% to 10.2% for the balloons compared with 3.3% to 3.4% with sham.[57–60]

Aspiration Therapy

The AspireAssist device was approved in 2016 for patients with a BMI of 35 to 55 kg/m^2.[61] It consists of a percutaneous gastrostomy tube, which is placed endoscopically and attached to an external aspiration port positioned at the abdominal surface. After each meal, patients aspirate approximately 30% of ingested food. AspireAssist is associated with 12.1% TBWL compared with 3.5% with lifestyle counseling alone.[62]

Hydrogel Capsules

Plenity is a capsule composed of cellulose and citric acid, which was approved in 2019 for patients with a BMI of 25 to 40 kg/m^2.[63] The superabsorbent hydrogel particles in the capsules absorb up to 100 times their weight in water and expand to occupy approximately a quarter of average stomach volume. Patients consume three capsules (2.25 g/dose) with water before lunch and dinner. Plenity is associated with 6.4% TBWL compared with 4.4% with placebo.[64]

TransPyloric Shuttle

The TransPyloric Shuttle is a device approved in 2019 for patients with a BMI of 25 to 40 kg/m^2.[65] It is comprised of a large spherical bulb connected to a small cylindrical weight. After endoscopic placement, an overtube facilitates coiling of a silicone cord into the bulb. The bulb remains above the pylorus to prevent migration out of the stomach while the weight moves freely in the duodenum. The TransPyloric Shuttle is associated with 9.5% TBWL compared with 2.8% with sham.[66]

Table 3
Devices approved for overweight and obesity by the FDA

Device	Description	Total Body Weight Loss (%)	FDA Approval
Orbera Intragastric Balloon[55]	Endoscopically placed intragastric balloon filled with 400–700 mL saline, removed endoscopically after 6 mo	10.2 Sham: 3.3 6 mo[57,58]	2015 BMI 30–40 kg/m²
Obalon Balloon System[56]	Three sequentially swallowed balloons each filled with 250 mL of gas, removed endoscopically 6 mo after first balloon placed	6.6 Sham: 3.4 6 mo[59,60]	2016 BMI 30–40 kg/m²
AspireAssist[61]	Endoscopically placed percutaneous gastrostomy aspiration tube; up to 30% of each meal removed from the stomach	12.1 Lifestyle alone:3.5 12 mo[62]	2016 BMI 35–55 kg/m²
Plenity[63]	Capsules containing superabsorbent hydrogel particles, which occupy a quarter of stomach volume when hydrated; three capsules (2.25 g/dose) administered with water before lunch and dinner	6.4 Placebo: 4.4 6 mo[64]	2019 BMI 25–40 kg/m²
TransPyloric Shuttle[65]	Endoscopically placed device comprised of a large spherical bulb (remains above pylorus) attached to a small cylindrical weight (moves freely in duodenum); removed endoscopically after 12 mo	9.5 Sham: 2.8 12 mo[66]	2019 BMI 30–40 kg/m²

Abbreviation: lifestyle, lifestyle counseling (diet + exercise).

SUMMARY

Weight management is an essential part of the treatment plan for patients with OSA and overweight or obesity because weight loss can lead to significant improvements in AHI. Lifestyle interventions including diet, physical activity, and behavioral modifications are the cornerstones of weight management; however, most patients have difficulty maintaining weight loss without advanced therapy. Health care providers who treat patients with OSA should be familiar with pharmacotherapy, surgery, and device options for patients with overweight and obesity. Because combination treatment can lead to additive or synergistic weight loss, the future of weight management is a customized, multidisciplinary approach for each patient.

DISCLOSURE

Dr K.H. Saunders and Dr L.I. Igel have an ownership interest in Intellihealth. Dr L.I. Igel is a consultant for Novo Nordisk. Dr B.G. Tchang has nothing to disclose.

REFERENCES

1. Young T, Peppard PE, Taheri S. Excess weight and sleep-disordered breathing. J Appl Physiol (1985) 2005;99(4):1592–9.
2. Gileles-Hillel A, Kheirandish-Gozal L, Gozal D. Biological plausibility linking sleep apnoea and metabolic dysfunction. Nat Rev Endocrinol 2016;12(5):290–8.

3. Joosten SA, Hamilton GS, Naughton MT. Impact of weight loss management in OSA. Chest 2017;152(1):194–203.

4. Peppard PE, Young T, Palta M, et al. Longitudinal study of moderate weight change and sleep-disordered breathing. JAMA 2000;284(23):3015–21.

5. Mitchell LJ, Davidson ZE, Bonham M, et al. Weight loss from lifestyle interventions and severity of sleep apnoea: a systematic review and meta-analysis. Sleep Med 2014;15(10):1173–83.

6. Foster GD, Borradaile KE, Sanders MH, et al. A randomized study on the effect of weight loss on obstructive sleep apnea among obese patients with type 2 diabetes: the Sleep AHEAD study. Arch Intern Med 2009;169(17):1619–26.

7. Johansson K, Hemmingsson E, Harlid R, et al. Longer term effects of very low energy diet on obstructive sleep apnoea in cohort derived from randomised controlled trial: prospective observational follow-up study. BMJ 2011;342:d3017.

8. Tuomilehto HP, Seppä JM, Partinen MM, et al. Lifestyle intervention with weight reduction: first-line treatment in mild obstructive sleep apnea. Am J Respir Crit Care Med 2009;179(4):320–7.

9. Buchwald H, Avidor Y, Braunwald E, et al. Bariatric surgery: a systematic review and meta-analysis. JAMA 2004;292(14):1724–37.

10. Dong Z, Hong BY, Yu AM, et al. Weight loss surgery for obstructive sleep apnoea with obesity in adults: a systematic review and meta-analysis protocol. BMJ Open 2018;8(8):e020876.

11. Drager LF, Brunoni AR, Jenner R, et al. Effects of CPAP on body weight in patients with obstructive sleep apnoea: a meta-analysis of randomised trials. Thorax 2015;70(3):258–64.

12. Tachikawa R, Ikeda K, Minami T, et al. Changes in energy metabolism after continuous positive airway pressure for obstructive sleep apnea. Am J Respir Crit Care Med 2016;194(6):729–38.

13. Chirinos JA, Gurubhagavatula I, Teff K, et al. CPAP, weight loss, or both for obstructive sleep apnea. N Engl J Med 2014;370(24):2265–75.

14. Dansinger ML, Gleason JA, Griffith JL, et al. Comparison of the Atkins, Ornish, weight watchers, and zone diets for weight loss and heart disease risk reduction: a randomized trial. JAMA 2005;293(1):43–53.

15. Hall KD, Ayuketah A, Brychta R, et al. Ultra-processed diets cause excess calorie intake and weight gain: an inpatient randomized controlled trial of ad libitum food intake. Cell Metab 2019;30(1):67–77.e3.

16. Lennerz BS, Alsop DC, Holsen LM, et al. Effects of dietary glycemic index on brain regions related to reward and craving in men. Am J Clin Nutr 2013;98(3):641–7.

17. Estruch R, Ros E, Salas-Salvadó J, et al. Primary prevention of cardiovascular disease with a Mediterranean diet. N Engl J Med 2013;368(14):1279–90.

18. Estruch R, Ros E, Salas-Salvadó J, et al. Primary prevention of cardiovascular disease with a Mediterranean diet supplemented with extra-virgin olive oil or nuts. N Engl J Med 2018;378(25):e34.

19. US Department of Health and Human Services. Physical activity guidelines for Americans. Available at: https://health.gov/paguidelines/. Accessed August 23, 2019.

20. Igel LI, Kumar RB, Saunders KH, et al. Practical use of pharmacotherapy for obesity. Gastroenterology 2017;152(17):30142–7.

21. Saunders KH, Igel LI, Shukla AP, et al. Drug-induced weight gain: rethinking our choices. J Fam Pract 2016;65(11):780–8.

22. Sumithran P, Prendergast LA, Delbridge E, et al. Long-term persistence of hormonal adaptations to weight loss. N Engl J Med 2011;365(17):1597–604.
23. Greenway FL. Physiological adaptations to weight loss and factors favouring weight regain. Int J Obes (Lond) 2015;39(8):1188–96.
24. Fothergill E, Guo J, Howard L, et al. Persistent metabolic adaptation 6 years after "The Biggest Loser" competition. Obesity (Silver Spring) 2016;24(8):1612–9.
25. Rosenbaum M, Leibel RL. Adaptive thermogenesis in humans. Int J Obes (Lond) 2010;34:S47–55.
26. Jensen MD, Ryan DH, Apovian CM, et al. 2013 AHA/ACC/TOS guideline for the management of overweight and obesity in adults: a report of the American College of Cardiology/American Heart Association Task Force on Practice Guidelines and the Obesity Society. J Am Coll Cardiol 2014;63(25 Pt B):2985–3023.
27. Apovian CM, Aronne LJ, Bessesen DH, et al. Pharmacological management of obesity: an Endocrine Society clinical practice guideline. J Clin Endocrinol Metab 2015;100(2):342–62.
28. Saunders KH, Umashanker D, Igel LI, et al. Obesity pharmacotherapy. Med Clin North Am 2018;102(1):135–48.
29. Saunders KH, Shukla AP, Igel LI, et al. Obesity: when to consider medication. J Fam Pract 2017;66(10):608–16.
30. Saunders KH, Kumar RB, Igel LI, et al. Pharmacologic approaches to weight management: recent gains and shortfalls in combating obesity. Curr Atheroscler Rep 2016;18(7):36.
31. Thomas CE, Mauer EA, Shukla AP, et al. Low adoption of weight loss medications: a comparison of prescribing patterns of antiobesity pharmacotherapies and SGLT2s. Obesity (Silver Spring) 2016;24(9):1955–61.
32. Aronne LJ, Wadden TA, Peterson C, et al. Evaluation of phentermine and topiramate versus phentermine/topiramate extended-release in obese adults. Obesity (Silver Spring) 2013;21(11):2163–71.
33. Adipex [package insert]. Tulsa (OK): Physicians Total Care, Inc; 2012.
34. Lomaira [package insert]. Newtown (PA): KVK-TECH, INC; 2016.
35. Kushner RF. Weight loss strategies for treatment of obesity. Prog Cardiovasc Dis 2014;56(4):465–72.
36. Gadde KM, Allison DB, Ryan DH, et al. Effects of low-dose, controlled-release, phentermine plus topiramate combination on weight and associated comorbidities in overweight and obese adults (CONQUER): a randomised, placebo controlled, phase 3 trial. Lancet 2011;377(9774):1341–52.
37. Qsymia [package insert]. Mountain View (CA): VIVUS, Inc; 2012.
38. Qsymia risk evaluation and mitigation strategy (REMS). VIVUS, Inc. Available at: http://www.qsymiarems.com/. Accessed August 23, 2019.
39. Greenway FL, Whitehouse MJ, Guttadauria M, et al. Rational design of a combination medication for the treatment of obesity. Obesity (Silver Spring) 2009; 17(1):30–9.
40. Greenway FL, Fujioka K, Plodkowski RA, et al. Effect of naltrexone plus bupropion on weight loss in overweight and obese adults (COR-I): a multicentre, randomised, double-blind, placebo-controlled, phase 3 trial. Lancet 2010;376(9741):595–605.
41. Contrave [package insert]. La Jolla (CA): Orexigen Therapeutics, Inc; 2016.
42. Pi-Sunyer X, Astrup A, Fujioka K, et al. A randomized, controlled trial of 3.0 mg of liraglutide in weight management. N Engl J Med 2015;373(1):11–22.
43. Saxenda [package insert]. Plainsboro (NJ): Novo Nordisk; 2014.
44. Marso SP, Daniels GH, Brown-Frandsen K, et al. Liraglutide and cardiovascular outcomes in type 2 diabetes. N Engl J Med 2016;375(4):311–22.

45. Torgerson JS, Hauptman J, Boldrin MN, et al. XENical in the prevention of diabetes in obese subjects (XENDOS) study: a randomized study of orlistat as an adjunct to lifestyle changes for the prevention of type 2 diabetes in obese patients. Diabetes Care 2004;27(1):155–61.
46. Xenical [package insert]. South San Francisco (CA): Genentech USA, Inc; 2015.
47. Alli [package insert]. Moon Township (PA): GlaxoSmithKline Consumer Healthcare, LP; 2015.
48. Lee JH, Nguyen QN, Le QA. Comparative effectiveness of 3 bariatric surgery procedures: Roux-en-Y gastric bypass, laparoscopic adjustable gastric band, and sleeve gastrectomy. Surg Obes Relat Dis 2016;12:997–1002.
49. Barenbaum SR, Saunders KH, Igel LI, et al. Obesity: when to consider surgery. J Fam Pract 2018;67(10):614, 616;618;620.
50. Colquitt JL, Pickett K, Loveman E, et al. Surgery for weight loss in adults. Cochrane Database Syst Rev 2014;(8):CD003641.
51. Heymsfield SB, Wadden TA. Mechanisms, pathophysiology, and management of obesity. N Engl J Med 2017;376:254–66.
52. Courcoulas AP, King WC, Belle SH, et al. Seven-year weight trajectories and health outcomes in the Longitudinal Assessment of Bariatric Surgery (LABS) Study. JAMA Surg 2018;153:427–34.
53. Roux CW, Heneghan HM. Bariatric surgery for obesity. Med Clin North Am 2018; 102:165–82.
54. Saunders KH, Igel LI, Saumoy M, et al. Devices and endoscopic bariatric therapies for obesity. Curr Obes Rep 2018;7(2):162–71.
55. Orbera intragastric balloon [package insert]. Austin (TX): Apollo Endosurgery; 2015.
56. Obalon balloon system [package insert]. Carlsbad (CA): Obalon Therapeutics, Inc.; 2016.
57. Courcoulas A, Abu Dayyeh BK, Eaton L, et al. Intragastric balloon as an adjunct to lifestyle intervention: a randomized controlled trial. Int J Obes (Lond) 2017;41(3):427–33.
58. U.S. Food and Drug Administration. PMA P140008: FDA summary of safety and effectiveness data. Available at: https://www.accessdata.fda.gov/cdrh_docs/pdf14/P140008b.pdf. Accessed August 23, 2019.
59. Sullivan S, Swain JM, Woodman G, et al. The Obalon swallowable 6-month balloon system is more effective than moderate intensity lifestyle therapy alone: results from a 6-month randomized sham controlled trial. Gastroenterology 2016;150(4 Suppl 1):S1267.
60. PMA P160001: FDA summary of safety and effectiveness data. Available at: https://www.accessdata.fda.gov/cdrh_docs/pdf16/P160001b.pdf. Accessed August 23, 2019.
61. AspireAssist [package insert]. King of Prussia (PA): Aspire Bariatrics; 2016.
62. Thompson CC, Abu Dayyeh BK, Kushner K, et al. The AspireAssist is an effective tool in the treatment of class II and class III obesity: results of a one-year clinical trial. Gastroenterology 2016;4(Suppl 1):S86.
63. Plenity [package insert]. Boston (MA): Gelesis, Inc; 2019.
64. Greenway FL, Aronne LJ, Raben A, et al. A randomized, double-blind, placebo-controlled study of Gelesis100: a novel nonsystemic oral hydrogel for weight loss. Obesity (Silver Spring) 2019;27(2):205–16.
65. TransPyloric Shuttle [package insert]. San Carlos (CA): BAROnova, Inc.; 2019.
66. U.S. Food and Drug Administration. PMA P180024: FDA summary of safety and effectiveness data. Available at: https://www.accessdata.fda.gov/cdrh_docs/pdf18/P180024B.pdf. Accessed August 23, 2019.

Palatopharyngoplasty and Palatal Anatomy and Phenotypes for Treatment of Sleep Apnea in the Twenty-first Century

Ryan Puccia, MD[a],*, Beverly Tucker Woodson, MD[b]

KEYWORDS

- Sleep apnea • Palate surgery • Pharyngoplasty • Expansion sphincterplasty

KEY POINTS

- The goal of palatopharyngoplasty is to open and stiffen the retropalatal airspace and lateral pharyngeal walls.
- The described modification allows for better stiffening and repositioning of the lateral pharyngeal wall, relocation of the palatopharyngeus muscles, and opening the retropalatal airway at the palatal genu.
- Removal of lateral palatal fat combined with a medial incision of the dorsal palatal mucosa creates a lateral and superior based flap (dorsal palatal flap) that provides improved control over tension on the lateral pharyngeal closure.

INTRODUCTION

Obstructive sleep apnea (OSA) is characterized by repeated apnea/hypoventilation with desaturation during sleep. The long-term significance and prevalence of this disease has been well documented and studied. Although continuous positive airway pressure (CPAP) therapy remains the gold standard, there remains a large group of individuals who are unable to tolerate this intervention. The most common surgical approach for OSA is the uvulopalatopharyngoplasty (UPPP).[1] As we discuss in this article, the surgical procedure has transformed significantly since its origin. This is in large part due to a better understanding of the functional anatomy and critically

[a] Department of Otolaryngology and Human Communication, Medical College Wisconsin, Milwaukee, WI 53226, USA; [b] Division of Sleep Medicine and Sleep Surgery, Department of Otolaryngology and Human Communication, Medical College Wisconsin, 98701 Watertown Plank Road, Milwaukee, WI 53226, USA
* Corresponding author.
E-mail address: rpuccia@mcw.edu

Otolaryngol Clin N Am 53 (2020) 421–429
https://doi.org/10.1016/j.otc.2020.02.005
0030-6665/20/Published by Elsevier Inc.

reviewing the characteristics of responders and nonresponders. As the field of sleep surgery expands and new procedures are being created to address the dynamic upper airway, a thorough understanding of the fundamental principles of this surgery is critical to success.

When it comes to surgical treatment of OSA, maxillomandibular advancement (MMA) is widely accepted as the most successful upper airway reconstructive procedure. Meta-analysis of limited case series supports a success rate of 86% and surgical cure of 43% with studies also demonstrating long-term success in high-risk, obese patients with severe disease.[2–4] Historically, such high success rates are attributed to its larger impact on "multilevel" upper airway obstruction in patients with sleep apnea. Although there is still much to learn about why surgeries are successful or failures, a remarkable body of evidence is beginning to support that the high success rates of MMA surgery is not due to elimination of obstruction in the lower pharyngeal airway and retroglossal airspace, but due to its effect on the upper pharynx and retropalatal airway.[3] Some have even referred to the procedure as a "skeletal palatopharyngoplasty." If MMA is but a better UPPP, then what are the overlapping features that we can learn to apply to UPPP surgery? One consistent finding on endoscopy for postoperative patients with MMA is demonstration of improvement in lateral wall stiffness.[4] Without changing the bony confines of the facial skeleton, we can change the paradigm of surgery from altering upper airway to not simply allow more room but to stiffen the lateral wall to minimize the dynamic collapse. This plays in to the evolution of the surgery through the years.

Initially, UPPP as described by Fujita was primarily an excisional technique with variable results. The main goal to was remove the tonsils, truncate the soft palate and uvula, and perform a pillarplasty.[5] Initially, there was a striking gap between those who responded well to surgery versus those who did not. Friedman and colleagues[6] was able to characterize these groups based on palate position and Brodsky tonsil size. Although success rates are high for adults with large tonsils (Friedman stage 1), success for unfavorable Friedman stage 3 (small tonsils) may be as low as 8%. Because of this, Browaldh and colleagues[7,8] gathered a cohort referred to as the Sleep Apnea Karolinska UPPP randomized controlled trial (SKUP3 RTC), which randomized 65 Friedman stage 1 and 2 patients into a treatment versus nontreatment control arm. They demonstrated significant improvements in Epworth sleepiness scale, physical and mental component scores on the short form-36 questionnaire, and increased sleep latency/vigilance testing.[7,8] The technique was a modification of Fujita's UPPP with a cold steel tonsillectomy and less extensive excision of the palate and tonsillar pillars. Although this demonstrated efficacy in individuals with favorable anatomy, there was still the question of how to surgically address the unfavorable Friedman 3 group. As mentioned previously, this required a change in paradigm from simply trying to create room by removing tissue to address specific anatomic components of the upper airway. In 2003, Cahali[9] described a modification of UPPP he called the lateral pharyngoplasty in an effort to address the collapsing lateral pharyngeal walls. In this procedure, the tonsils were removed to expose the superior pharyngeal constrictor within the fossa. The muscle was then elevated and sectioned in a craniocaudle direction, generating 2 muscle flaps. The lateral flap was then sutured anteriorly to the palatoglossus. He also made superior palatal wedge incisions to identify the superior aspect of the palatopharyngeus, which was fully sectioned and sutured in a z-plastylike fashion to the palate. Although this demonstrated promising results, patients experienced significant postoperative dysphagia. In 2007, Pang and Woodson[10] proposed the expansion sphincterplasty based on work by Orticochea and Christel (who developed a palatopharyngeal sphincter by apposition of these muscles). This modification of the lateral pharyngoplasty procedure took care to leave the superior constrictor intact but transected the palatopharyngeus low and sutured this anterolaterally on the palate to expand the retropalatal space (**Figs. 1** and **2**). The cohort that this surgery was specifically trying to address was the Friedman stage 3 anatomy and those with lateral pharyngeal wall collapse. They randomized 45 patients into the expansion sphincterplasty group and traditional UPPP group and found superior results with expansion sphincterplasty in this cohort.[10] Although there are numerous other modifications described, the overarching trend is away from traditional excisional UPPP and toward modified versions that aim to target and exploit the regional anatomy. The lead author of this article has further modified the technique, which is discussed later in this article in current practice.

It is worth noting that the success rate of palate surgery for OSA is widely variable, and in some studies has been reported as low as 40% to 50% in unselected patients.[11] This is complicated by numerous factors, including definitions of surgical success, surgical cure, and differences in objective polysomnography. Classically, surgical success defined by Sher and colleagues[11] is 50% reduction in Apnea-Hypopnea Index (AHI) and AHI level less than 20. Some advocate for a surgical cure defined by a postoperative AHI less than 10.[12] Some studies have looked at the difference in success rates comparing various forms of palate surgeries, and although limited in number and inability to show significance, expansion sphincterplasty trended toward superior results.[12] Results by Pang and Woodson[10] comparing expansion sphincterplasty with traditional UPPP in all Friedman groups indicated success rates of 82% for expansion compared with 68% for traditional. Interestingly, despite wide ranges in objective AHI improvement, patients subjectively feel better. Validated sleep-related quality of life questionnaires at 3 and 6 months postoperatively from palate surgery have been studied and consistently demonstrate improved quality of life in surgical groups.[13] Although reported results are variable in the literature, and it is important to critically appraise definitions of success, there is clearly a population that responds better to UPPP than others.

Much research has gone into predicting who will respond well to UPPP. Although the Friedman staging system is useful, what else should clinicians be looking for to determine candidacy? Other variables thought to be a negative predictor of success include low hyoid position.[14] This is likely because a low hyoid relates to a longer upper airway, which is flow limiting based on the Poiseuille equation. Age, body mass index (BMI), and preoperative AHI have not been found to be predictors of UPPP outcomes.[14–16] As described previously, reconstructive techniques, such as

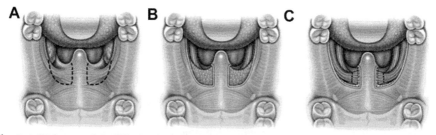

Fig. 1. Initial steps of modified expansion sphincterplasty are shown. Ventral palatal mucosa and lateral palatal fat are removed (*A*). Removal is superficial to muscles but aggressively removes ventral fat. Midline mucosa is preserved for creation of new "neo-uvula" (*B*). Palatoglossus muscle. is incised medially and removed exposing palatopharyngeus muscle and superior constrictor muscles (*C*). (*Courtesy of* B Tucker Woodson, MD, Milwaukee, WI.)

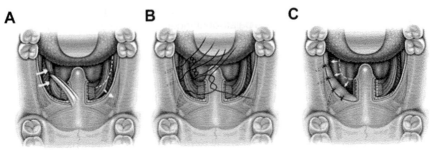

Fig. 2. Palatopharyngeus Muscle. is bluntly dissected from superior constrictor from a level of the velopharynx proximal to the limits of exposure. Multiple veins may need bipolar cautery and care is made to not violate the superior constrictor and expose parapharyngeal fat laterally nor to violate the nasopharyngeal mucosa medially (A). Right arrow indicates cut and self retracted palatoglossus muscle. Left arrows indicate mobilized palatopharyngeous muscle mobilized off the constrictor. Three sutures are "slung" around the palatopharyngeus muscle to expand the pharynx laterally, superiorly, and anteriorly. Sutures are anchored to the fascia around the hamulus[1] and to the pterygomandibular raphe laterally[2] (B). After muscle lateralization, the dorsal palatal mucosa is incised immediately adjacent to the uvula muscle, creating a dorsal palatal flap. This flap, which is based laterally and superiorly, is then closed to the ventral palatal mucosa. Raw surface of the uvula is left to heal secondarily. In some patients, a limited excision of the distal tip of the new "neouvula" is conservatively excised (C). Arrows indicate the rolled dorsal palatal flap for mucosal closure. (*Courtesy of* B Tucker Woodson, MD, Milwaukee, WI.)

expansion pharyngoplasty and other modified procedures, demonstrate improvements over classic UPPP; however, technical failures remain an issue.

Preoperative evaluation for pharyngoplasty continues to evolve. Traditional radiographic, office-based, or endoscopic techniques have been replaced by Drug Induced Sleep Endoscopy (DISE). The traditional VOTE classification created a systematic language to assess the common points of collapse in the upper airway.[17] Although it was able to create a common language, it remains controversial in many ways. First, the ideal drug for sedation is unclear, and although it does parallel natural sleep, they are not the same.[18,19] Although propofol is a common choice, dosing and protocols are numerous and may impact the airflow changes seen even in sleep. Second, the impact of using DISE on overall outcomes has been debated with mixed results in the literature. In 2019, Green and colleagues[19] published the first multicenter trial looking at the impact of DISE on surgical outcomes. A total of 275 patients over 14 centers were included. DISE interpretations were blinded, although interestingly, interrater reliability was only moderate even in an experienced group of readers. Looking at AHI reduction as a primary outcome measure, 2 groups distinctly performed worse in this cohort: those with oropharyngeal lateral wall collapse and those with complete tongue base collapse. Outside of the traditional VOTE criteria, as understanding of the anatomy and airflow mechanics has improved, we can better apply the information from DISE to critically appraise patient-specific anatomy in the preoperative evaluation. In this regard, phenotypes of the soft palate have been described. Of note is the angle of the soft palate at the anatomic genu, which is defined by the tensor veli palatini. This angle has been described as the alpha angle and is of importance when understanding postoperative failure proximal to the surgical site.[20] An alpha angle that is large, indicating an obtuse-angled palate, is more favorable for UPPP, as there will be less retropalatal narrowing above the surgical expansion. An acute angle is likely to have a narrow anterior-posterior gap above the surgical site and is a well-known site of failure in UPPP surgery.[20,21]

With regard to preoperative evaluation, another emerging technology in assessment of the upper airway is Computational Fluid Dynamics. This technique uses a computed tomography image captured with patients in supine position, jaw in normal occlusion, and in a nasal inspiratory phase. These data are then constructed into a 3-dimensional rendering of the patient's upper airway where modeling can be used to estimate flow and model flow restriction at the level of the retro palatal and retroglossal airway.[22] Although not mainstream, reduction in retropalatal airflow velocity has been demonstrated in postoperative MMA patients.[22]

When considering the tenets of reconstructive surgery, form and function must be taken into account. Variations of rearrangement of the muscular slings in the throat are limited by the other functions. In this light, complications of surgery also must be considered. One big consideration in postoperative UPPP patients is the safety and efficacy of their swallow. Patients with OSA tend to have subclinical deficits in swallow function postoperatively with noted hypopharyngeal stasis and laryngeal penetration.[23] Studies indicate that many of the postoperative changes tend to resolve by a month after surgery.[24] Some of these changes include a prolonged hyoid movement time that further increases the risk of hypopharyngeal stasis and laryngeal penetration. Decreased movement of the velum and decreased pharyngeal constriction time were also noted postoperatively, which returned to normal within a month.[24] One important consideration for the cause of these changes is the loss of oropharyngeal sensibility in addition to the manipulation of the oropharyngeal musculature. Other studies have demonstrated an increase in the upper esophageal sphincter (UES) tone on manometry in postoperative patients and increased hypopharyngeal bolus pressures possibly due to the changes in oropharyngeal sensation leading to loss of ability to fully relax the UES.[23] Because the current technique may alter lateral wall and palate movement more than prior techniques, a specific screening for swallowing dysfunction may be indicated.

The history of the UPPP procedure demonstrates significant evolution over time. The preoperative workup from physical examination, Friedman staging, low hyoid positioning, and endoscopic examination evaluating for multilevel collapse, integrity of the lateral walls, and the nature/angle and length of the genu are all important in the assessment of candidacy for successful UPPP. This evolution in patient selection and surgical philosophy is driven in large part by a better understanding of the anatomy and history of treatment for patients with OSA.

ANATOMY AND PHYSIOLOGY OF OBSTRUCTIVE SLEEP APNEA AS RELATES TO PALATE SURGERY

The anatomy of the soft palate is complex. The conglomerate action of numerous muscle slings in physiologic motion is not fully understood. Although anatomy texts describe the individual muscle relationships, they do not consider the dynamic and various forces created with many muscles working at once. Cadaver studies are limited in availability, cultural differences, and unknown presence or absence of sleep apnea physiology and anatomy.[25] A better understanding of not only the dynamic anatomy, but variation and patient-specific components may increase successful UPPP selection.

The soft palate contains a ventral (oral) surface that is primarily fibrofatty in nature. The dorsal (nasal) surface of the palate contains the denser fascia that unites with the hard palate and aponeurosis of the various soft palate muscles, which are described as follows.

The tensor veli palatini (TVP) is a muscular sling that originates on the anterior aspect of the eustachian tube cartilage, wraps around the hamulus inferiorly, and then inserts onto the aponeurosis of the soft palate. This muscle defines the anatomic genu of the soft palate. As discussed previously, this muscle is the defining point of the alpha angle and the transition to the descending portion of the palate should be noted in length and slope.

The levator veli palatini is a related muscular sling that originates posterior on the eustachian tube cartilage and extends into the soft palate aponeurosis.

The palatoglossus (PG) is a thin and small muscular contribution which extends from the palate to the tongue. This muscle is not robust and will likely not anchor the denser muscles posterior forward but will likely be pulled posteriorly by the more robust musculature.

The palatopharyngeus (PP) is of particular importance, typically described as having 3 muscle bundles: a dorsal, ventral, and transverse. The transvers bundle extends circumferentially around the superior constrictor to create a sphincterlike effect. This thickening is historically referred to as the Passavant ridge or a thickening of the superior constrictor itself.

The superior constrictor muscle is the final sling that houses the upper airway around the velum. This muscle extends circumferentially, forming the back wall of the airway and the lateral walls as it inserts into the pterygomandibular raphe anteriorly and the hyoid bone inferiorly. Of note, the muscularis uvulae is an intrinsic muscle of the soft palate present within the uvular tip.[25]

CURRENT TECHNIQUE

The following is a description of the current UPPP technique used by BTW.

After the mouth gag is placed, the surgical landmarks are identified. These include the hamulus on both sides of the palate, the pterygomandibular raphe, and the dimple point that is determined with where the soft palate collapses when it is flexed by grasping the uvula. Wedge incisions are then planned from the superior tonsillar pillar to 4 to 5 mm anterior on the soft palate from the apex of the dimple point; 1% lidocaine with 1:100,000 epinephrine is then infiltrated into the operative site, and tonsillectomy is performed. After tonsillectomy, the ventral palatal wedge incisions are then made. Tissue is excised to the level of the muscle. The fibrofatty tissue of the ventral soft palate is extensively removed with attention to the removal of the lateral palatal fat. With the underlying palatal muscles exposed, the PG is usually released and self-retracts into the submucosa laterally.

The PP is then carefully dissected off the superior constrictor muscle. This can be done bluntly and/or with bipolar cautery, as a parapharyngeal venous plexus is sometimes encountered. This step is key to generate mobility off the constrictor so the muscle bundles can be pulled anterolaterally under less tension. It is important to be cognizant of not only violating the superior constrictor laterally to the parapharyngeal space but also not dissecting too deep and perforating the mucosa as it wraps posteriorly around the PP into the oropharynx. "Sling" sutures (three 2-0 Vicryls bilaterally) are then used to grab full-thickness sections of the mobilized PP muscle. The sutures of the superior region are anchored anterior and laterally to the dense aponeurosis around the hamulus as far in the apex of the palatal incision as possible. The sutures of the lower region are anchored to the pterygomandibular raphe. In a subgroup of patients, dissection of the PP off the superior constrictor is inadequate to relocate the PP to the anchoring point of the pterygomandibular raphe. In those patients, the PP muscle may be transected and mobilized, as in the traditional expansion pharyngoplasty procedure. The procedure concludes with the dorsal palatal flap for closure. This is accomplished with a full-thickness dorsal palatal incision adjacent to the uvula bilaterally. This reduces the sphincter action of the transverse PP bundle. These flaps are rotated and sewed over the deep layer, concluding the expansion pharyngoplasty.

FUTURE DIRECTIONS

One shortcoming of research in sleep surgery is current long-term data. This is due in part to various definitions of long term, heterogeneity of data, and techniques. One recent meta-analysis from 2018 looked at 59 papers over the past 17 years with 2715 patients who underwent palate surgery. Some interesting findings include a decrease in the percentage of classic UPPP surgery that is being implemented (25.67% from 2001 to 2010, to 12.6% from 2011 to 2018).[26] This is likely due to the change in paradigm discussed previously in favor of less excisional and more reconstructive targeted techniques. This also demonstrated that the AHI reduction in the expansion sphincterplasty was greater than classic UPPP. Another meta-analysis from 2019 looked at long-term efficacy defined as more than 34 months after surgery. Interestingly, long-term outcomes were still effective, although there was a decrease over time noted, with an average increase in AHI of 12.3 events per hour (63.8%) and a decrease in surgical response from 67.3% to 44.35%.[27] Even with this decrease in efficacy over time, there is still symptomatic improvement. Interestingly, predictors of long-term failure included patients with high BMI, low arterial oxygen saturations, and longer time with less than 90% oxygen saturation. This indicates those with more severe OSA or obesity may be more likely to lose surgical efficacy over time.[27]

Along these lines, surgical relapse remains a prominent concern. Surgical decision making for patients with OSA has become more complex with the expansion of techniques and anatomic understanding provided by DISE. Liu and colleagues[28] proposed the Stanford protocol to form a tiered approach to sleep surgery, which was recently revised in 2019. The revision focuses on a more comprehensive approach, including bariatric surgery for obese individuals, identification of upper airway subsite, and interventions to perform with promotion of MMA in cases of surgical relapse or treatment failure. As the anatomy is dynamic, however, changes made at time of surgery may alter the airflow dynamics that change the pattern of collapse in an entirely new way, which may be able to be addressed surgically.

With the advent of other techniques in upper airway surgery, such as upper airway stimulation (UAS), UPPP may be something to consider in an adjuvant role. In a recent article by Hasselbacher and colleagues,[29] 15 patients with complete concentric collapse (CCC) at the velum underwent UPPP with before and after DISE and PSG; 93% of patients (all but one) demonstrated a change in collapse pattern. Thirteen patients had persistent collapse at the velum (9 partial, 4 complete), 1 completely resolved, and 1 had persistent CCC. This is important in that CCC is currently a contraindication for UAS. Given the favorable results of UAS in the treatment of OSA for specific patient cohorts, resolving CCC may open other favorable therapeutic alternatives.

More information is needed to deepen our understanding of sleep surgery. The UPPP procedure has evolved significantly since its origin due to better understanding of the anatomy, the advent of endoscopy, and other surgical alternatives. For patients with multilevel collapse, multisite surgery is standard. Better understanding of how procedures at each level influence each other may be the next step in optimization. If the goal is to stiffen the airway to prevent dynamic collapse, techniques below and above the level of collapse may augment surgery at the level. Surgical alternatives may not be a one or the other style approach but may complement each other to promote overall and long-term efficacy. Because of this, the UPPP will continue to be a mainstay of sleep surgery moving into the future and will likely continue to evolve as new technology and understanding emerge.

DISCLOSURE

The authors have nothing to disclose.

REFERENCES

1. Stuck BA, Ravesloot MJ, Eschenhagen T, et al. Uvulopalatopharyngoplasty with or without tonsillectomy in the treatment of adult obstructive sleep apnea–a systematic review. Sleep Med 2018;50:152–65.
2. Liu SYC, Huon LK, Iwasaki T, et al. Efficacy of maxillomandibular advancement examined with drug-induced sleep endoscopy and computational fluid dynamics airflow modeling. Otolaryngol Head Neck Surg 2016;154(1):189–95.
3. Chang KK, Kim KB, McQuilling MW, et al. Fluid structure interaction simulations of the upper airway in obstructive sleep apnea patients before and after maxillomandibular advancement surgery. Am J Orthod Dentofacial Orthop 2018; 153(6):895–904.
4. Liu SYC, Huon LK, Powell NB, et al. Lateral pharyngeal wall tension after maxillomandibular advancement for obstructive sleep apnea is a marker for surgical success: observations from drug-induced sleep endoscopy. J Oral Maxillofac Surg 2015;73(8):1575–82.
5. Conway WA, Slcklesteel JM, Wittig RM, et al. Evaluation of the effectiveness of uvulopalatopharyngoplasty. Laryngoscope 1985;95(1):70–4.
6. Friedman M, Ibrahim H, Joseph NJ. Staging of obstructive sleep apnea/hypopnea syndrome: a guide to appropriate treatment. Laryngoscope 2004;114(3): 454–9.
7. Browaldh N, Bring J, Friberg D. SKUP 3 RCT; continuous study: changes in sleepiness and quality of life after modified UPPP. Laryngoscope 2016;126(6): 1484–91.
8. Browaldh N, Bring J, Friberg D. SKUP3: 6 and 24 months follow-up of changes in respiration and sleepiness after modified UPPP. Laryngoscope 2018;128(5): 1238–44.
9. Cahali MB. Lateral pharyngoplasty: a new treatment for obstructive sleep apnea hypopnea syndrome. Laryngoscope 2003;113(11):1961–8.
10. Pang KP, Woodson BT. Expansion sphincter pharyngoplasty: a new technique for the treatment of obstructive sleep apnea. Otolaryngol Head Neck Surg 2007; 137(1):110–4.
11. Sher AE, Schechtman KB, Piccirillo JF. The efficacy of surgical modifications of the upper airway in adults with obstructive sleep apnea syndrome. Sleep 1996; 19(2):156–77.
12. Carrasco-Llatas M, Marcano-Acuña M, Zerpa-Zerpa V, et al. Surgical results of different palate techniques to treat oropharyngeal collapse. Eur Arch Otorhinolaryngol 2015;272(9):2535–40.
13. Weaver EM, Woodson BT, Yueh B, et al, SLEEP Study Investigators. Studying Life Effects & Effectiveness of Palatopharyngoplasty (SLEEP) study: subjective outcomes of isolated uvulopalatopharyngoplasty. Otolaryngol Head Neck Surg 2011;144(4):623–31.

14. Choi JH, Cho SH, Kim SN, et al. Predicting outcomes after uvulopalatopharyng-oplasty for adult obstructive sleep apnea: a meta-analysis. Otolaryngol Head Neck Surg 2016;155(6):904–13.
15. Liao YF, Chuang ML, Huang CS, et al. Upper airway and its surrounding struc-tures in obese and nonobese patients with sleep-disordered breathing. Laryngo-scope 2004;114(6):1052–9.
16. Zhang J, Li Y, Cao X, et al. The combination of anatomy and physiology in pre-dicting the outcomes of velopharyngeal surgery. Laryngoscope 2014;124(7): 1718–23.
17. Kezirian EJ, Hohenhorst W, de Vries N. Drug-induced sleep endoscopy: the VOTE classification. Eur Arch Otorhinolaryngol 2011;268(8):1233–6.
18. Mahmoud M, Ishman SL, McConnell K, et al. Upper airway reflexes are preserved during dexmedetomidine sedation in children with Down syndrome and obstruc-tive sleep apnea. J Clin Sleep Med 2017;13(05):721–7.
19. Green KK, Kent DT, D'Agostino MA, et al. Drug-induced sleep endoscopy and surgical outcomes: a multicenter cohort study. Laryngoscope 2019;129(3): 761–70.
20. Woodson BT. A method to describe the pharyngeal airway. Laryngoscope 2015; 125(5):1233–8.
21. Woodson BT, Sitton M, Jacobowitz O. Expansion sphincter pharyngoplasty and palatal advancement pharyngoplasty: airway evaluation and surgical techniques. Oper Tech Otolayngol Head Neck Surg 2012;23(1):3–10.
22. Mihaescu M, Mylavarapu G, Gutmark EJ, et al. Large eddy simulation of the pharyngeal airflow associated with obstructive sleep apnea syndrome at pre and post-surgical treatment. J Biomech 2011;44(12):2221–8.
23. Schar M, Woods C, Ooi EH, et al. Pathophysiology of swallowing following oropharyngeal surgery for obstructive sleep apnea syndrome. Neurogastroen-terol Motil 2018;30(5):e13277.
24. Corradi AM, Valarelli LP, Grechi TH, et al. Swallowing evaluation after surgery for obstructive sleep apnea syndrome: uvulopalatopharyngoplasty vs. expansion pharyngoplasty. Eur Arch Otorhinolaryngol 2018;275(4):1023–30.
25. Cho JH, Kim JK, Lee HY, et al. Surgical anatomy of human soft palate. Laryngo-scope 2013;123(11):2900–4.
26. Pang KP, Plaza G, Reina COC, et al. Palate surgery for obstructive sleep apnea: a 17-year meta-analysis. Eur Arch Otorhinolaryngol 2018;275(7):1697–707.
27. He M, Yin G, Zhan S, et al. Long-term efficacy of uvulopalatopharyngoplasty among adult patients with obstructive sleep apnea: a systematic review and meta-analysis. Otolaryngol Head Neck Surg 2019;161(3):401–11.
28. Liu SYC, Awad M, Riley R, et al. The role of the revised stanford protocol in to-day's precision medicine. Sleep Med Clin 2019;14(1):99–107.
29. Hasselbacher K, Seitz A, Abrams N, et al. Complete concentric collapse at the soft palate in sleep endoscopy: what change is possible after UPPP in patients with CPAP failure? Sleep Breath 2018;22(4):933–8.

Base of Tongue Surgery for Obstructive Sleep Apnea in the Era of Neurostimulation

Ravi R. Shah, MD, Erica R. Thaler, MD*

KEYWORDS

- Obstructive sleep apnea • Base of tongue • Sleep surgery
- Transoral robotic surgery • Upper airway stimulation

KEY POINTS

- Proper characterization of a patient's airway collapse pattern is critical to selecting a successful surgical approach for treatment of obstructive sleep apnea.
- Procedures for base of tongue tissue reduction and repositioning include transoral robotic surgery, radiofrequency ablation, midline glossectomy, genioglossus advancement, hyoid suspension, and maxillary-mandibular advancement.
- With a single procedure, upper airway stimulation can improve retroglossal and retropalatal obstruction, adding to potential approaches to base of tongue collapse.
- Specific tongue base approaches may vary in response to patient and surgeon preferences and be used in multilevel surgery where appropriate.
- Key factors in deciding between upper airway stimulation and tongue base reduction include patient age, anatomic factors, body mass index, and willingness to undergo device implantation.

INTRODUCTION

For the large number of patients with obstructive sleep apnea (OSA) who fail or cannot tolerate positive pressure airway therapy, there are a spectrum of oral appliances and surgical procedures designed to relieve the causative anatomic obstruction.[1] However, airway obstruction can occur at multiple anatomic levels, and collapse patterns are highly variable from patient to patient.[2,3] Therefore, proper characterization of a patient's collapse pattern is critical to selecting a successful surgical approach.

In more than 70% of cases, the tongue base contributes to obstruction during sleep.[2] As a result, several surgical procedures have been developed to target tongue

Department of Otorhinolaryngology–Head and Neck Surgery, University of Pennsylvania, Hospital of the University of Pennsylvania, 3400 Spruce Street, 5th Floor Silverstein Building, Philadelphia, PA 19104, USA
* Corresponding author.
E-mail address: erica.thaler@uphs.upenn.edu

Otolaryngol Clin N Am 53 (2020) 431–443
https://doi.org/10.1016/j.otc.2020.02.006
0030-6665/20/© 2020 Elsevier Inc. All rights reserved.

base obstruction. Procedures include transoral robotic surgery (TORS) glossectomy, radiofrequency ablation (RFA) of the tongue, and midline glossectomy (with or without coblation).[4–12] Procedures that reposition the tongue include genioglossus advancement, hyoid suspension, and maxillary-mandibular advancement.[13–17] Upper airway stimulation (UAS) of the hypoglossal nerve also alleviates tongue base obstruction by dynamic stimulation of the genioglossus, causing tongue protrusion.[18,19]

Although procedures for tongue base debulking have been in use since the 1990s, UAS represents a fairly recent addition to the sleep surgeon's armamentarium and has decreased some of the need for surgeries directed solely at base of tongue obstruction.[20,21] With a single procedure, UAS can improve both retroglossal and retropalatal obstruction.[22,23] However, ablative surgeries are still widely used in a multilevel approach, and maxillary-mandibular advancement addresses multiple levels of obstruction as well.[6,17,24] Furthermore, candidacy limitations, variable anatomy, refractory sleep apnea, and both patient and surgeon preferences still leave room for select roles for base of tongue surgery in the treatment of OSA.

We discuss major elements that guide patient selection for various surgical approaches to tongue base resection for OSA, with special attention to the growing role of UAS.

TRANSORAL ROBOTIC SURGERY

TORS has been used successfully for the treatment of OSA since 2009, approximately 5 years before UAS was approved for OSA.[5,19,20] Vicini and colleagues[5] first published their preliminary results on TORS for patients with OSA primarily owing to tongue base hypertrophy in 2010, where they demonstrated feasibility of TORS for tongue base resection as well as epiglottoplasty. Soon after in 2012, Lee and colleagues[6] published their early data in a prospective trial using TORS as part of a multilevel approach to sleep apnea surgery. In this study, patients underwent uvulopalatopharyngoplasty as well as TORS-assisted partial glossectomy, which is notable in that UAS also addresses collapse at the levels of both the palate and tongue base. Importantly, and unlike the patient population for which UAS has been tested, there were no maximum limits on body mass index (BMI) or Apnea-Hypopnea Index (AHI) in the study by Lee and associates.[6]

Although there are no randomized controlled prospective comparisons between TORS and UAS, the 2 approaches have been compared in retrospective studies.[20,21] Although both approaches demonstrated superior results for UAS, both studies also showed significant roles for TORS in select patients.

Yu and colleagues[20] reviewed candidacy criteria for TORS, including drug-induced sleep endoscopy videos of 152 patients who had TORS during the period when UAS was not yet approved. Of the 152, 20 would have met candidacy criteria for UAS based on BMI, AHI, and drug-induced sleep endoscopy findings of anteroposterior collapse (**Fig. 1**). These patients were compared with 27 patients who had undergone UAS by the time of the study who also met TORS candidacy criteria, namely, retroglossal collapse. This study had 2 major conclusions. First, patients who underwent UAS had more dramatic improvements in objective measures of OSA compared with patients who underwent TORS: AHI reduction was 12.7 for TORS patients compared with 33.3 for UAS patients, and the cure rate (AHI <5) was 10.0% for TORS versus 70.3% for UAS (**Table 1**). However, 78.2% of the 152 patients who underwent TORS did not meet AHI and BMI criteria for UAS, and 86.8% did not meet all AHI, BMI, and drug-induced sleep endoscopy criteria for UAS. This study clearly illustrated the continued need for TORS in select patients with sleep apnea.

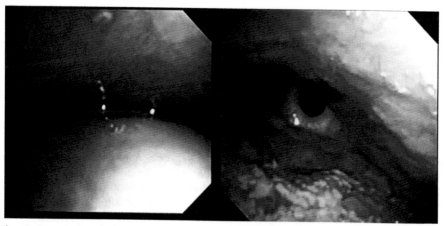

Fig. 1. Drug-induced sleep endoscopy at both the retropalatal and retroglossal levels showing anteroposterior collapse in a TORS patient who would have qualified for UAS surgery. (*From* Yu JL, Mahmoud A, Thaler ER. Transoral robotic surgery versus upper airway stimulation in select obstructive sleep apnea patients. Laryngoscope. 2019;129(1):256–8; with permission.)

Huntley and colleagues[21] also showed greater improvement in patients who underwent UAS compared with TORS in a review of patients over a 6.5-year period from 2011 to 2017. Postoperative AHI and O_2 nadir improved to 20.1% and 84.1%, respectively, for TORS patients compared with 7.2% and 88.8% for UAS patients. Additionally, a decrease in the AHI to less than 5 was 20.8% for TORS versus 59.2% for UAS. Although both TORS and UAS were available for approximately one-half of the study period and a selection bias may have been present, the authors noted that UAS largely replaced TORS at their institution. Still, the authors stated that they continue to use TORS "in patients who are found to have lingual tonsil hypertrophy contributing to their obstruction." Furthermore, they found age to be a significant difference between TORS and UAS patients, with TORS patients being on average significantly younger (46.4 years) compared with UAS patients (61.9 years; $P<.001$).

These studies bring to light important considerations in patient selection for TORS versus UAS. One of the most obvious is the candidacy limitations on UAS. UAS, specifically the Inspire II implant (Inspire Medical Systems, Inc, Maple Grove, MN), is approved for patients 22 years of age or older, with an AHI of 15 to 65, and who do not have complete concentric collapse of the soft palate, among other criteria.[25]

Table 1
Results of study showing significant differences in reduction of AHI, percent of sleep time with an oxygen saturation of less than 90% (SaO_2 <90%), oxygen nadir, and cure rate

	TORS	UAS	P Value
Average AHI reduction	12.7	33.3	.002
Average change SaO_2 <90%	1.30%	14.1	.02
Average change in O_2 nadir	2.60%	12.10%	<.001
Cure rate	10.00%	70.40%	<.001

From Yu JL, Mahmoud A, Thaler ER. Transoral robotic surgery versus upper airway stimulation in select obstructive sleep apnea patients. Laryngoscope. 2019;129(1):256–8; with permission.

Additionally, the device has mostly been tested in patients with a BMI of less than 35.[19] MRI can only be performed of the head and extremities with certain conditions in patients who have Inspire Model 3028, and MRI cannot be performed at all in patients with Inspire Model 3024.[25] TORS notably has none of these limitations. However, it must be stated that although there is no BMI limit for TORS, patients with a BMI of greater than 40 tend not to do as well as patients with a BMI of 30 to 40, who in turn do not do as well as patients with a BMI of less than 30.[26]

With regards to patient anatomy, UAS is not an option for patients with concentric collapse or predominantly lateral collapse, whereas TORS often still is.[20,25] Moreover, although both UAS and TORS can improve obstruction at the levels of both the palate and tongue base, TORS also allows management of epiglottic collapse. Although there is case report evidence of UAS improving epiglottic collapse, substantial evidence is lacking, and the current body of literature supports repositioning or resection to successfully manage epiglottic obstruction.[27–29] The transoral robotic approach provides excellent access for epiglottopexy or partial epiglottectomy for patients with significant epiglottic prolapse into the larynx.[30]

In addition, patient and surgeon preferences and risk tolerances factor into the equation. As Huntley and coworkers[21] observed, patients who undergo TORS tend to be younger. This circumstance may be due to a combination of younger patients being more hesitant to undergo implantation of a device and possibly surgeons implicitly being more reluctant to implant younger patients. Additional considerations are the differences inherent to the nature of the techniques, namely, differences in postoperative course and potential complications. Patients who undergo TORS typically are admitted to the hospital for overnight observation, whereas UAS is performed as an outpatient surgery. Postoperative restrictions differ; for TORS, diet is restricted to initial nil per os or liquid diet with gradual advancement as tolerated beginning on postoperative day 1, whereas for UAS, the arm on the implanted side is kept in a sling for 48 hours.[23,31] Complications of TORS include transient tongue numbness, taste disturbance, dysphagia, edema potentially necessitating overnight intubation or reintubation, and oropharyngeal bleeding potentially requiring cauterization (**Table 2**).[26,32] By contrast, complications of UAS include tongue discomfort, tongue abrasions from dental contact, transient tongue weakness, surgical site complications at any of the 3 incisions (scar, numbness, wound dehiscence, hematoma, and surgical site infection), pneumothorax, insomnia, device infection, and device failure potentially requiring surgery to remove or exchange the device.[19,33–35]

For qualifying patients who fail prior airway surgery, UAS can still be offered. As shown initially by Mahmoud and colleagues[36] and subsequently by g and colleagues[37] using the ADHERE Registry, prior airway surgery has no statistically significant impact on UAS efficacy. Conversely, of the 37% of patients who fail UAS, tongue base resection via TORS or an alternate approach may be an option in appropriate patients.[33]

RADIOFREQUENCY ABLATION

RFA, which has been used for various medical and surgical applications since the 1970s, is another technique that has been adapted for the treatment of OSA.[7,38,39] Radiofrequency is on the lowest end of the electromagnetic frequency spectrum and can thus deliver energy to deep tissue at relatively low temperatures.[9] The energy delivered to tissue by specially designed probes causes coagulation necrosis, inflammation, and subsequent fibrosis in the targeted tissue, with limited effect on surrounding structures.[9] Powell and colleagues first described the use of RFA for tongue base ablation in 1999 (**Fig. 2**). Patients received an average of 10 treatments over a mean of

Table 2 Surgical complications	
Complication Type	**n**
Bleeding	12
Dehydration requiring treatment	14
Dysphagia/odynophagia requiring treatment	15
Pneumonia	6
Reintubation	2
>6-Hour intubation	2
Hypoxemia	6
Pain[a]	3
Gastrointestinal complications	1
Cardiac arrhythmias	1
Other[b]	15
Total	77[c]

[a] Types of pain included chest pain, throat pain, and unspecified pain.
[b] Other complications included nausea, deep venous thrombosis, urinary retention, shortness of breath, tongue swelling, atelectasis, aspiration pneumonitis, thrush, encephalopathy, superficial venous thrombophlebitis, fever, possible transient ischemic attack, altered mental status, bronchitis, and orthostatic hypotension.
[c] There were 77 total complications in 59 patients.
From Hoff PT, D'Agostino MA, Thaler ER. Transoral robotic surgery in benign diseases including obstructive sleep apnea: Safety and feasibility. Laryngoscope. 2015;125(5):1249–53; with permission.

5.5 sessions, with a mean of 8490 J delivered. Postoperative MRI demonstrated a 17% decrease in preoperative tongue volume after an initial 10.8% increase at 24 to 48 hours owing to edema.[7] Impressively, the Respiratory Disturbance Index (RDI) was reduced by 55% and O_2 nadir improved from 81.9% to 88.1% on average at a mean follow-up time of 17 weeks.

Over the years, variations on the technique emerged, including multilevel RFA of the palate in addition to the tongue base. Additionally, Steward and colleagues[8] showed that additional treatments correlated with improved outcomes in 2004. A 2008 meta-analysis by Farrar and colleagues[9] corroborated the efficacy of RFA on short-term follow-up, with a mean 31% decrease in RDI for results at or within 12 months, but the study also exposed a paucity of long-term data, noting only 2 studies followed patients beyond 2 years.[40,41]

Although there have been no direct comparisons between RFA and UAS, RFA has shown smaller improvements relative to TORS in both subjective and objective outcomes. A randomized controlled trial by Woodson and colleagues[42] showed an apnea index reduction but not an AHI reduction, suggesting a shift of apneic events to hypopneic events without complete resolution of these respiratory disturbances. In meta-analyses, compared with the 31% RDI reduction for RFA, TORS has demonstrated a 60% reduction in AHI. Furthermore, compared with the 31% reduction in the Epworth Sleepiness Scale for RFA, TORS has demonstrated a 55% decrease.[9,26] Admittedly, this oversimplifies the comparison, because patient selection as well as other confounders may factor into the individual studies within these 2 completely separate meta-analyses. However, it gets to the root of the question of patient selection criteria for TORS versus RFA. Although results are more modest and cure rate may be lower, RFA is a minimally invasive, less painful procedure with a quicker recovery relative to

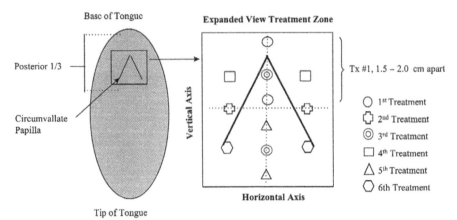

Fig. 2. Treatment zone of base of tongue. Treatment zone is 2.5 to 3.0 cm² and circumscribes the circumvallate papilla. Treatment distance between each lesion site is 1.5 to 2.0 cm apart (eg, treatment 1 [Tx #1]). Two treatment sites (radiofrequency lesions) are given during a treatment session and are spaced as shown in the figure. Treatment sites alternate between the vertical and horizontal axes of the tongue until the final treatment is given. (*From* Powell NB, Riley RW, Guilleminault C. Radiofrequency tongue base reduction in sleep-disordered breathing: A pilot study. Otolaryngol Head Neck Surg. 1999;120(5):656–64; with permission.)

TORS.[43] An important distinction between RFA and other tongue base surgeries is that RFA may require multiple sessions.[44] Finally, many of the potential complications are minor, but RFA is still an airway surgery with the risk for potential airway compromise. The spectrum of complications of RFA includes vasovagal syncope, lingual nerve hypesthesia, hypoglossal nerve paresis, odynophagia, floor of mouth hematoma, mucosal ulceration, tongue base cellulitis and/or abscess in some cases requiring tracheostomy, and tongue edema requiring hospitalization (**Table 3**).[9,44]

Therefore, RFA may be an appropriate option for patients seeking minimal pain and rapid recovery for moderate results. Patient preferences may weigh in more heavily when considering RFA versus UAS, because UAS is likely to have superior results based on the present data, but patients may opt to avoid device implantation.[9,19,34,44,45] Furthermore, as stated elsewhere in this article, UAS can be offered for patients with OSA refractory to other surgical procedures without significant impact on efficacy.[36,37]

MIDLINE GLOSSECTOMY AND COBLATION

There are numerous additional techniques for tongue base resection for the treatment of OSA, many of which are modifications of the midline glossectomy originally described by Dorrity and colleagues[10,44] in 1991. Small studies and wide institutional variations render comprehensive analysis difficult, but pivotal techniques and considerations are discussed.

Fujita and associates[10] first demonstrated success with midline glossectomy in 1991 using a CO_2 laser. In this approach, a mouth gag was used for the anterior portion of the dissection, followed by microdirect laryngoscopy for the tongue base. In addition to tongue base resection, Fujita and coworkers reported performing aryepiglottic fold reduction and partial epiglottectomy when appropriate. Of the 12 patients

Table 3 Complications of RFA in the OSA patient population	
Tongue Base RFA Complications	**Events (252 Patients over 1092 Treatment Sessions), n (%)**
Floor of mouth hematoma	8 (0.7)
Tongue cellulitis w/o abscess	7 (0.6)
Tongue edema requiring hospitalization	7 (0.6)
Mucosal ulceration	6 (0.6)
Tongue base abscess	3 (0.3)
Hypoglossal nerve paresis	3 (0.3)
Lingual nerve hypesthesia	2 (0.2)
Prolonged odynophagia	1 (0.1)
Vasovagal syncope	1 (0.1)
Total	38 (3.5)

Adapted from Farrar J, Ryan J, Oliver E, Gillespie MB. Radiofrequency ablation for the treatment of obstructive sleep apnea: a meta-analysis. Laryngoscope. 2008;118(10):1878–83; with permission.

studied, 11 had failed prior uvulopalatopharyngoplasty. Five patients (42%) had a significant decrease in their RDI, from a mean of 60.6 to 14.5. These patients had lower BMI relative to the nonresponders (30.6 vs 37.9) and tended to be more retrognathic on cephalometric analysis. Complications included minor bleeding, prolonged odynophagia, and dysgeusia.[10]

Woodson and Fujita[46] extended this procedure to include lingualplasty 1 year after describing the initial midline glossectomy. After performing the initial midline glossectomy, Woodson and Fujita[46] described excising bilateral wedges of tongue tissue adjacent to the midline resection, then suturing the wedges closed by bringing posterior tissue anteriorly, resulting in a T-shaped closure (**Fig. 3**). Tracheostomy was performed in most patients before glossectomy. In this group, 17 of 22 patients with severe OSA had a significant reduction in RDI, from a mean of 58.8 to 8.1. Complications were similar to the isolated midline glossectomy, with the addition of tongue edema in 1 patient and subcutaneous emphysema related to tracheostomy in 1 patient. Although no clear distinction could be made between responders and nonresponders, overall, the results seemed to be more promising than midline glossectomy alone.[46] In both variations of the procedure, patients were admitted postoperatively with a liquid diet beginning on postoperative day 1 and thereafter advanced as tolerated.

Glossectomy using other instruments and approaches have also been described. The use of plasma wand tools, namely a Coblator (Smith & Nephew, London, UK), a submucosal approach to the tongue base via incision in the oral tongue and endoscopic visualization, and additional lateral resection channels in addition to the midline resection have all been described with some degree of success in case series.[11,12,44,47]

Robinson and colleagues[11] first used a bipolar radiofrequency plasma wand to perform submucosal tongue base resection with ultrasound guidance in 15 patients in 2003. Their results are difficult to ascribe solely to the tongue base resection, because 2 patients had mucosal suture advancement of the tongue base, patients with coexisting retropalatal collapse had concurrent uvulopalatopharyngoplasty, and 5 of the 15 patients had additional palatal advancement and hyoid suspension.

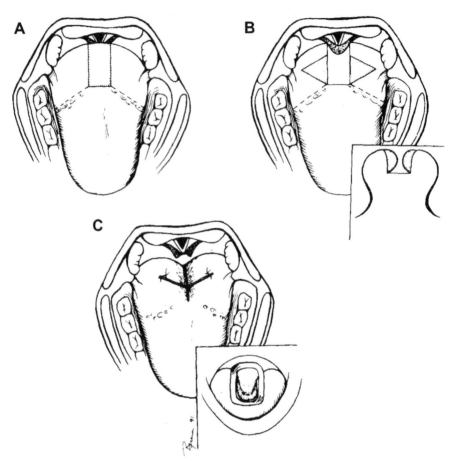

Fig. 3. Lingualplasty is performed by, first, excision of a midline segment of tongue poste-rior to the circumvallate papillae (*A*). The prolapsing tissue (*B*) is then excised in a wedge shape (*B, inset*). Posterior tissue is then sutured anteriorly (*C*). Partial epiglottectomy is shown (*C, inset*). (*From* Woodson BT, Fujita S. Clinical experience with lingualplasty as part of the treatment of severe obstructive sleep apnea. Otolaryngol Head Neck Surg. 1992;107(1):40–8; with permission.)

Still, their initial results demonstrated a 40% success rate, defined as a more than 50% decrease in RDI and achieving an RDI of less than 20. Twelve of the patients were kept intubated postoperatively for several hours. There were 3 major complications, which included hematoma requiring emergent tracheostomy, wound infection, and tempo-rary hypoglossal nerve neuropraxia.[11]

Notably, Maturo and Mair[12] successfully treated OSA in 3 pediatric patients with macroglossia using a plasma wand with endoscopic visualization and ultrasound guidance via their submucosal minimally invasive lingual excision approach (**Fig. 4**). There were no infection or bleeding events postoperatively. Additionally, although their initial patients were kept intubated prophylactically overnight, Maturo and Mair[12] dis-cussed that there was no significant tongue base edema and in their later patients they began extubating postoperatively.[12]

Consideration of midline glossectomy and/or lingualplasty techniques compared with other tongue base resection approaches may vary by institution and surgeon

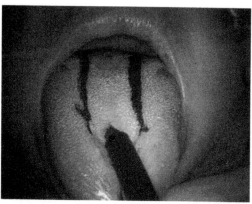

Fig. 4. An EVac 70 T&A Plasma Wand is placed inside tongue through anterior submucosal incision. Tactile palpation (along with ultrasonography and endoscopy) ensures relatively safe tongue base tissue removal. (*From* Maturo SC, Mair EA. Submucosal minimally invasive lingual excision: an effective, novel surgery for pediatric tongue base reduction. Ann Otol Rhinol Laryngol. 2006;115(8):624–30; with permission.)

preference. For example, surgeons may prefer laser or coblation owing to decreased heat and depth of penetration of tissue damage, theoretically resulting in less postoperative pain compared with traditional electrocautery in, for example, a TORS approach. With respect to coblation, recent studies show statistically similar polysomnographic outcomes between TORS and coblation, with perhaps slightly better results using TORS.[43,48,49] However, coblation has a lower rate of minor complications, a quicker return to normal diet, and a lower cost compared with TORS.[43,49] However, the idea of decreased pain with coblation remains controversial in the tonsillectomy literature, where it has been best studied.[50–53] The level of invasiveness of the midline glossectomy variations and potential complications remain roughly the same as with TORS; therefore, selection between midline glossectomy versus UAS involves largely the same thought process between patient and surgeon.

The main difference is in the success of endoscopic lingual tonsillectomy and posterior midline glossectomy in pediatric patients, a demographic in which TORS has not been well-studied.[54] Regardless of the approach, tongue base reduction or repositioning techniques are typically offered before UAS, because the use of UAS has not yet been approved in patients younger than 22 years.[25,54] However, the role of UAS is in pediatrics is evolving: Diercks and colleagues[27,55] reported initial success implanting a hypoglossal nerve stimulator in an adolescent with Down syndrome and severe, refractory OSA requiring tracheostomy. Additionally, Caloway and Diercks more recently demonstrated safety and efficacy of UAS in a case series of 20 patients with Down syndrome and severe OSA aged 10 to 21 years.[27,55]

SUMMARY

Retroglossal collapse is commonly seen in patients with OSA. The role of UAS for these patients continues to evolve. However, base of tongue reduction surgery continues to have usefulness for appropriately selected patients with OSA. Selection of a specific tongue base approach may vary in response to both patient and surgeon preferences, and the tongue base approach can be used in a multilevel approach where appropriate. Key factors include patient age, willingness to undergo device implantation, and preferences for outpatient versus inpatient procedure, single procedure versus multiple, and tolerance for various procedure-specific postoperative restrictions and potential complications.

DISCLOSURE

The authors have nothing to disclose.

REFERENCES

1. Weaver TE, Sawyer AM. Adherence to continuous positive airway pressure treatment for obstructive sleep apnoea: implications for future interventions. Indian J Med Res 2010;131:245–58.
2. Kezirian EJ, White DP, Malhotra A, et al. Interrater reliability of drug-induced sleep endoscopy. Arch Otolaryngol Head Neck Surg 2010;136(4):393–7.
3. Charakorn N, Kezirian EJ. Drug-induced sleep endoscopy. Otolaryngol Clin North Am 2016;49(6):1359–72.
4. O'Malley BW Jr, Weinstein GS, Snyder W, et al. Transoral robotic surgery (TORS) for base of tongue neoplasms. Laryngoscope 2006;116(8):1465–72.
5. Vicini C, Dallan I, Canzi P, et al. Transoral robotic tongue base resection in obstructive sleep apnoea-hypopnoea syndrome: a preliminary report. ORL J Otorhinolaryngol Relat Spec 2010;72(1):22–7.
6. Lee JM, Weinstein GS, O'Malley BW Jr, et al. Transoral robot-assisted lingual tonsillectomy and uvulopalatopharyngoplasty for obstructive sleep apnea. Ann Otol Rhinol Laryngol 2012;121(10):635–9.
7. Powell NB, Riley RW, Guilleminault C. Radiofrequency tongue base reduction in sleep-disordered breathing: a pilot study. Otolaryngol Head Neck Surg 1999; 120(5):656–64.
8. Steward DL, Weaver EM, Woodson BT. A comparison of radiofrequency treatment schemes for obstructive sleep apnea syndrome. Otolaryngol Head Neck Surg 2004;130(5):579–85.
9. Farrar J, Ryan J, Oliver E, et al. Radiofrequency ablation for the treatment of obstructive sleep apnea: a meta-analysis. Laryngoscope 2008;118(10):1878–83.
10. Fujita S, Woodson BT, Clark JL, et al. Laser midline glossectomy as a treatment for obstructive sleep apnea. Laryngoscope 1991;101(8):805–9.
11. Robinson S, Lewis R, Norton A, et al. Ultrasound-guided radiofrequency submucosal tongue-base excision for sleep apnoea: a preliminary report. Clin Otolaryngol Allied Sci 2003;28(4):341–5.
12. Maturo SC, Mair EA. Submucosal minimally invasive lingual excision: an effective, novel surgery for pediatric tongue base reduction. Ann Otol Rhinol Laryngol 2006;115(8):624–30.
13. Riley R, Guilleminault C, Powell N, et al. Mandibular osteotomy and hyoid bone advancement for obstructive sleep apnea: a case report. Sleep 1984;7(1):79–82.
14. Riley RW, Powell NB, Guilleminault C. Inferior sagittal osteotomy of the mandible with hyoid myotomy-suspension: a new procedure for obstructive sleep apnea. Otolaryngol Head Neck Surg 1986;94(5):589–93.
15. Hormann K, Baisch A. The hyoid suspension. Laryngoscope 2004;114(9): 1677–9.
16. Riley RW, Powell NB, Guilleminault C, et al. Maxillary, mandibular, and hyoid advancement: an alternative to tracheostomy in obstructive sleep apnea syndrome. Otolaryngol Head Neck Surg 1986;94(5):584–8.

17. Riley RW, Powell NB, Guilleminault C. Obstructive sleep apnea syndrome: a surgical protocol for dynamic upper airway reconstruction. J Oral Maxillofac Surg 1993;51(7):742–7 [discussion: 748–9].

18. Eisele DW, Smith PL, Alam DS, et al. Direct hypoglossal nerve stimulation in obstructive sleep apnea. Arch Otolaryngol Head Neck Surg 1997;123(1):57–61.

19. Woodson BT, Soose RJ, Gillespie MB, et al. Three-year outcomes of cranial nerve stimulation for obstructive sleep apnea: the STAR trial. Otolaryngol Head Neck Surg 2016;154(1):181–8.

20. Yu JL, Mahmoud A, Thaler ER. Transoral robotic surgery versus upper airway stimulation in select obstructive sleep apnea patients. Laryngoscope 2019; 129(1):256–8.

21. Huntley C, Topf MC, Christopher V, et al. Comparing upper airway stimulation to transoral robotic base of tongue resection for treatment of obstructive sleep apnea. Laryngoscope 2019;129(4):1010–3.

22. Safiruddin F, Vanderveken OM, de Vries N, et al. Effect of upper-airway stimulation for obstructive sleep apnoea on airway dimensions. Eur Respir J 2015;45(1): 129–38.

23. Heiser C, Thaler E, Boon M, et al. Updates of operative techniques for upper airway stimulation. Laryngoscope 2016;126(Suppl 7):S12–6.

24. Thaler ER, Schwab RJ. Single-institution experience and learning curve with upper airway stimulation. Laryngoscope 2016;126(Suppl 7):S17–9.

25. Inspire Sleep Apnea Innovation - Indications/Contraindications. Available at: https://professionals.inspiresleep.com/indications-contridications/. Accessed August 9, 2019.

26. Miller SC, Nguyen SA, Ong AA, et al. Transoral robotic base of tongue reduction for obstructive sleep apnea: a systematic review and meta-analysis. Laryngoscope 2017;127(1):258–65.

27. Diercks GR, Keamy D, Kinane TB, et al. Hypoglossal nerve stimulator implantation in an adolescent with down syndrome and sleep apnea. Pediatrics 2016; 137(5) [pii:e20153663].

28. Heiser C. Advanced titration to treat a floppy epiglottis in selective upper airway stimulation. Laryngoscope 2016;126(Suppl 7):S22–4.

29. Torre C, Camacho M, Liu SY, et al. Epiglottis collapse in adult obstructive sleep apnea: a systematic review. Laryngoscope 2016;126(2):515–23.

30. Thaler E. Chapter 54: management of the epiglottis. In: Friedman M, Jacobowitz O, editors. Sleep apnea and snoring: surgical and non-surgical therapy. 2nd edition. New York: Elsevier; 2019. p. 311–4.

31. D'Agostino MA. Transoral robotic partial glossectomy and supraglottoplasty for obstructive sleep apnea. Otolaryngol Clin North Am 2016;49(6):1415–23.

32. Hoff PT, D'Agostino MA, Thaler ER. Transoral robotic surgery in benign diseases including obstructive sleep apnea: safety and feasibility. Laryngoscope 2015; 125(5):1249–53.

33. Strollo PJ Jr, Soose RJ, Maurer JT, et al. Upper-airway stimulation for obstructive sleep apnea. N Engl J Med 2014;370(2):139–49.

34. Green KK, Woodson BT. Upper airway stimulation therapy. Otolaryngol Clin North Am 2016;49(6):1425–31.

35. Arteaga AA, Pitts KD, Lewis AF. Iatrogenic pneumothorax during hypoglossal nerve stimulator implantation. Am J Otolaryngol 2018;39(5):636–8.

36. Mahmoud AF, Thaler ER. Upper airway stimulation therapy and prior airway surgery for obstructive sleep apnea. Laryngoscope 2018;128(6):1486–9.

37. Kezirian EJ, Heiser C, Steffen A, et al. Previous surgery and hypoglossal nerve stimulation for obstructive sleep apnea. Otolaryngol Head Neck Surg 2019; 161(5):897–903.

38. Sweet WH, Wepsic JG. Controlled thermocoagulation of trigeminal ganglion and rootlets for differential destruction of pain fibers. 1. Trigeminal neuralgia. J Neurosurg 1974;40(2):143–56.

39. LeVeen HH, Wapnick S, Piccone V, et al. Tumor eradication by radiofrequency therapy. Responses in 21 patients. JAMA 1976;235(20):2198–200.

40. Li KK, Powell NB, Riley RW, et al. Temperature-controlled radiofrequency tongue base reduction for sleep-disordered breathing: long-term outcomes. Otolaryngol Head Neck Surg 2002;127(3):230–4.

41. Steward DL, Weaver EM, Woodson BT. Multilevel temperature-controlled radiofrequency for obstructive sleep apnea: extended follow-up. Otolaryngol Head Neck Surg 2005;132(4):630–5.

42. Woodson BT, Steward DL, Weaver EM, et al. A randomized trial of temperature-controlled radiofrequency, continuous positive airway pressure, and placebo for obstructive sleep apnea syndrome. Otolaryngol Head Neck Surg 2003;128(6): 848–61.

43. Friedman M, Hamilton C, Samuelson CG, et al. Transoral robotic glossectomy for the treatment of obstructive sleep apnea-hypopnea syndrome. Otolaryngol Head Neck Surg 2012;146(5):854–62.

44. Dorrity J, Wirtz N, Froymovich O, et al. Genioglossal advancement, hyoid suspension, tongue base radiofrequency, and endoscopic partial midline glossectomy for obstructive sleep apnea. Otolaryngol Clin North Am 2016;49(6):1399–414.

45. Wray CM, Thaler ER. Hypoglossal nerve stimulation for obstructive sleep apnea: a review of the literature. World J Otorhinolaryngol Head Neck Surg 2016;2(4): 230–3.

46. Woodson BT, Fujita S. Clinical experience with lingualplasty as part of the treatment of severe obstructive sleep apnea. Otolaryngol Head Neck Surg 1992; 107(1):40–8.

47. MacKay SG, Jefferson N, Grundy L, et al. Coblation-assisted Lewis and MacKay operation (CobLAMO): new technique for tongue reduction in sleep apnoea surgery. J Laryngol Otol 2013;127(12):1222–5.

48. Hwang CS, Kim JW, Kim JW, et al. Comparison of robotic and coblation tongue base resection for obstructive sleep apnoea. Clin Otolaryngol 2018;43(1):249–55.

49. Cammaroto G, Montevecchi F, D'Agostino G, et al. Tongue reduction for OSAHS: TORSs vs coblations, technologies vs techniques, apples vs oranges. Eur Arch Otorhinolaryngol 2017;274(2):637–45.

50. Parsons SP, Cordes SR, Comer B. Comparison of posttonsillectomy pain using the ultrasonic scalpel, coblator, and electrocautery. Otolaryngol Head Neck Surg 2006;134(1):106–13.

51. Hasan H, Raitiola H, Chrapek W, et al. Randomized study comparing postoperative pain between coblation and bipolar scissor tonsillectomy. Eur Arch Otorhinolaryngol 2008;265(7):817–20.

52. Wilson YL, Merer DM, Moscatello AL. Comparison of three common tonsillectomy techniques: a prospective randomized, double-blinded clinical study. Laryngoscope 2009;119(1):162–70.

53. Parker D, Howe L, Unsworth V, et al. A randomised controlled trial to compare postoperative pain in children undergoing tonsillectomy using cold steel dissection with bipolar haemostasis versus coblation technique. Clin Otolaryngol 2009; 34(3):225–31.

54. Ishman SL, Chang KW, Kennedy AA. Techniques for evaluation and management of tongue-base obstruction in pediatric obstructive sleep apnea. Curr Opin Otolaryngol Head Neck Surg 2018;26(6):409–16.
55. Caloway CL, Diercks GR, Keamy D, et al. Update on hypoglossal nerve stimulation in children with down syndrome and obstructive sleep apnea. Laryngoscope 2019. https://doi.org/10.1002/lary.28138.

Implantable Neurostimulation for Treatment of Sleep Apnea

Present and Future

Rachel Whelan, MD[a], Ryan J. Soose, MD[b],*

KEYWORDS

- Obstructive sleep apnea • Upper airway stimulation • Hypoglossal nerve stimulation
- Neurostimulation

KEY POINTS

- In contrast to traditional site-specific surgical procedures, hypoglossal nerve stimulation (HNS) offers the potential to address the multilevel airway collapsibility that is often involved in obstructive sleep apnea (OSA) without altering upper airway anatomy.
- At present, HNS therapy is considered second-line therapy for patients with moderate to severe OSA who are intolerant or unable to achieve adequate adherence with positive pressure therapy and who meet specific clinical, polysomnographic, and anatomic screening criteria.
- With the current available HNS system, detailed understanding of hypoglossal neuroanatomy is critical to optimal cuff electrode placement. Meticulous inclusion of tongue protrusor branches (genioglossus activation) with exclusion of tongue retractor branches (styloglossus and hyoglossus) sets the foundation for robust tongue protrusion.
- Data from the STAR trial, post-market institutional studies, and the multicenter ADHERE registry support clinically meaningful improvements in both objective and patient-reported outcome measures, favorable therapy adherence, and low perioperative risk across populations intolerant of continuous positive airway pressure.

INTRODUCTION

A growing understanding of the global prevalence of obstructive sleep apnea (OSA) and the impact of untreated OSA on neurocognitive function, quality of life, public

[a] Department of Otolaryngology, University of Pittsburgh School of Medicine, UPMC Mercy, University of Pittsburgh, Suite 2100, 1400 Locust Street, Pittsburgh, PA 15219, USA; [b] Division of Sleep Surgery, Department of Otolaryngology, University of Pittsburgh School of Medicine, UPMC Mercy, University of Pittsburgh, Suite 2100, 1400 Locust Street, Pittsburgh, PA 15219, USA
* Corresponding author.
E-mail address: sooserj@upmc.edu

Otolaryngol Clin N Am 53 (2020) 445–457
https://doi.org/10.1016/j.otc.2020.02.007
0030-6665/20/© 2020 Elsevier Inc. All rights reserved.

health and safety, and cardiovascular morbidity and mortality have driven a concomitant need for novel therapeutic options. Although positive airway pressure (PAP) therapy has substantial outcomes data for decades and remains the standard first-line treatment for most patients with OSA, particularly with more severe disease, many patients remain unable or unwilling to adhere to PAP therapy. To that end, well-designed trials with close clinical monitoring and advanced troubleshooting techniques demonstrate that PAP adherence rates remain suboptimal.[1-3]

Similarly, mandibular repositioning device (MRD) therapy has established itself as a robust first-line or second-line treatment; however, lack of adequate dentition, device-related side effects, and/or incomplete therapy response may preclude long-term use for many patients. Recent longitudinal studies demonstrate that at least half of MRD patients will develop occlusal changes that often necessitate discontinuation of therapy.[4] Moreover, traditional pharyngeal and skeletal reconstructive surgical treatments have limitations in long-term outcomes as well as limitations in applicability and acceptance across large populations, at least in part due to the potential postoperative side effects, morbidity, and risk.[5-7] As multilevel upper airway collapsibility is a hallmark of disease for many patients, it is not surprising that site-specific surgical options oftentimes fall short.

Over the past decade, hypoglossal nerve stimulation (HNS) therapy has emerged as a hybrid *surgically implanted* yet *medically titratable* option to fill the preceding unmet need for at least a subset of the untreated OSA population. HNS is uniquely characterized as a surgical procedure that does not alter upper airway anatomy, in addition to being a medical device therapy that does not require wearing an external apparatus (which is the root of much of the nonadherence concerns associated with PAP and MRD therapies). HNS is now an established and robust treatment alternative for an anatomic and physiologic subset of patients with moderate to severe OSA who are intolerant or unable achieve benefit with PAP or other first-line treatments.

BACKGROUND
Scientific Rationale of Therapy

Although most patients with OSA have some degree of anatomic upper airway vulnerability driving the disease, a growing body of literature indicates that dysfunctional neuromuscular control of breathing during sleep also plays a key role in the pathophysiology of many patients with OSA.[8] The upper airway neuromuscular feedback control loop consists of an afferent pathway from the pharyngeal mucosa and superior laryngeal nerve, and an efferent pathway through the hypoglossal motor nerve to the genioglossus and other upper airway dilator muscles.[9] Whereas healthy non-OSA controls respond to negative intraluminal pressure with a corresponding increase in genioglossus electromyographic activity, patients with OSA have evidence of inadequate neuromuscular control mechanisms including abnormal tonic activity of the upper airway dilator muscles and abnormal hypoglossal nerve conduction studies.[10] Activating the efferent limb with electrical stimulation of the upper airway dilator muscles directly or via the hypoglossal nerve has therefore emerged as the therapeutic target for OSA management.

Animal and Human Basic Science Studies

Decades of animal and human basic science studies confirmed the feasibility of electrical stimulation of the hypoglossal nerve and the subsequent associated improvement in airflow and reduction in upper airway collapsibility.[11] Particularly because the hypoglossal nerve contains only motor fibers rather than sensory, electrical neurostimulation was also shown to be well-tolerated without pain or arousal from sleep. One key breakthrough in therapy development was the importance of selective nerve stimulation illustrated by Oliven and colleagues[12]: selective stimulation of the genioglossus branches only resulted in anterior displacement of the tongue with concomitant improved airflow and airway stability, whereas selective stimulation of the styloglossus and hyoglossus branches caused posterior displacement of the tongue and associated collapse of the upper airway.

As such, cadaveric studies detailing the distal neuroanatomy of the hypoglossal nerve and functional muscle anatomy of the human tongue were critical to the development of the current surgical technique and electrode placement.[13,14] Selectively activating the terminal branches responsible for upper airway dilation while excluding all retractor branches appears to provide optimal tongue motion and outcomes with the currently available commercial system. Although the topography and number of distal nerve branches vary among individuals, the overall branching pattern remains consistent and predictable with genioglossus and geniohyoid branches arising from the medial aspect of the nerve.[15]

Another key finding in the early therapy development was the fact that stimulation of the hypoglossal nerve had the potential to provide a *multilevel* upper airway effect. In contrast to traditional single-site tongue base surgeries, upper airway endoscopy and imaging studies showed that selective neurostimulation resulted in enlargement and stabilization of not only the retrolingual portion of the airway but also the retroepiglottic and retropalatal spaces[16] (**Fig. 1**).

KEY CLINICAL STUDIES
Pilot and Feasibility Studies

Following the first human pilot study in 2001, multiple investigators and medical device companies spent a decade improving on the technology and studying their devices in larger trials. Eastwood and colleagues[17] (n = 21) and Kezirian and colleagues[18] (n = 31) studied the Hypoglossal Nerve Stimulation System (Apnex Medical, Inc., St. Paul, MN) and showed significantly reduced mean apnea-hypopnea index (AHI) at 6 and 12 months, respectively, with reported adverse events including a combined total of 2 infections requiring device removal and 3 cuff electrode dislodgements. Mwenge and colleagues[19] (n = 14) studied the Aura6000 System (ImThera Medical, Inc., San Diego, CA), which consists of a cuff electrode that is continuously activated

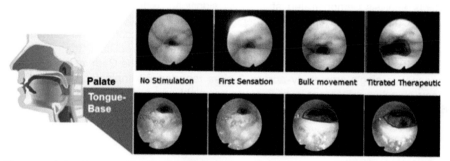

Fig. 1. Multilevel upper airway effect of HNS. Due in part to the mechanical coupling of the tongue and soft palate, increasing stimulation amplitude results not only in incremental enlargement of the retrolingual portion of the upper airway but also enlargement of the retropalatal airway. (Image courtesy of Inspire Medical Systems.)

and therefore does not require a respiratory sensor. Results demonstrated a significant improvement in mean AHI at 12 months, with reported adverse events including 2 participants with transient tongue paresis. Van de Heyning and colleagues[20] studied the Inspire II UAS System (Inspire Medical Systems, Inc., Maple Grove, MN) in an initial feasibility study that identified AHI less than 50 events per hour, body mass index (BMI) $\leq$32 kg/m^2, and absence of complete concentric pattern of palatal collapse on drug-induced sleep endoscopy (DISE) as predictors of response to therapy.

Pivotal Stimulation Therapy for Apnea Reduction Trial

The pivotal Stimulation Therapy for Apnea Reduction (STAR) trial incorporated these findings from the feasibility study into the pivotal trial inclusion criteria. The STAR trial was a multicenter prospective observational cohort study with a randomized withdrawal arm at 12 months.[21] After clinical, polysomnographic, and anatomic screening, 126 continuous PAP (CPAP)-intolerant participants, with moderate-severe OSA (AHI 20–50), BMI $\leq$32 kg/m^2, and absence of a complete concentric palatal collapse on DISE, underwent device implantation. Patient-reported and polysomnography outcome measures were assessed at regular intervals across a 5-year follow-up.

The 12-month primary (AHI, 4% oxygen desaturation index [ODI]) and secondary (Epworth Sleepiness Scale [ESS], Functional Outcomes of Sleep Questionnaire [FOSQ]) all demonstrated statistically significant improvement, and self-reported nightly adherence was 86%.[21] No changes in tongue function or morphology were identified and serious postsurgical adverse events were rare. The most common nonserious adverse event was therapy-related tongue soreness due to either the stimulation itself or tongue abrasion from an adjacent tooth. Reported data at the 24-month mark showed continued significant improvement in ESS and FOSQ scores and data at the 3- and 5-year marks further supported sustained long-term improvements in AHI as well as ESS and FOSQ scores.[22–24]

Post-Market Studies

After Food and Drug Administration (FDA) approval of the Inspire II system (Inspire Medical Systems, Inc. Maple Grove, MN) in 2014, outcomes from routine clinical practice continued to show high therapy adherence rates measured by objective device adherence monitoring, as well as objective improvements in OSA outcomes based on postoperative polysomnography that even exceeded STAR trial results, with an accompanying overall low rate of adverse events.[25] A metanalysis in 2015 included results from 6 prospective studies with 200 total patients. At 12 months, the pooled fixed effects analysis demonstrated statistically significant reductions in AHI, ODI, and ESS.[26] Comparison of outcomes of consecutive patients between independent academic institutions demonstrated remarkably consistent outcomes and adherence, suggesting that the therapy could be broadly translated and applicable to routine clinical practices, outside of a clinical trial setting.[27] Similarly, the German post-market prospective single-arm study across 3 sites reported 60 implanted patients with mean objective adherence over 6 hours per night and a median AHI reduction at 6 months from 28.6 to 8.3 events per hour.[28]

CLINICAL INDICATIONS AND CARE PATHWAY

A comprehensive sleep medicine history with upper airway phenotyping remains the cornerstone for the initial evaluation of all patients considering HNS therapy. Patients with hypoventilation syndromes or complex sleep-disordered breathing states due to chronic obstructive pulmonary disease, congestive heart failure, opioid medication, or other causes may not be suitable candidates. Similarly, significant sleep medicine comorbidities (eg, severe insomnia), physical limitations (eg, head and neck cancer, breast cancer reconstruction, or chest wall deformity), or imaging requirements (eg, MRI) may be relative contraindications to implantation.

Based on the available literature and FDA labeling, HNS therapy is considered second-line therapy for those patients with moderate to severe OSA (AHI between 15 and 65 events per hour) who have failed a trial of PAP therapy. Additional screening criteria currently include central and mixed apnea events comprising fewer than 25% of the total AHI and absence of a complete concentric pattern of palatal collapse on DISE. Significant obesity is a relative contraindication, depending on physician judgment and the remainder of the patient's anatomic and physiologic phenotype, with published guidelines currently ranging from $\leq$32 kg/m^2 to $\leq$35 kg/m^2. It is imperative to recognize, however, that although screening guidelines exist, patient selection must be determined on an individual basis within the broader clinical context of the patient's age, occupation, skeletal structure, pharyngeal anatomy, nasal airway, obesity and fat distribution, comorbid sleep disorders, medical and psychiatric comorbidities, OSA pathophysiology, and suitability for general anesthesia and surgical intervention.

The current clinical care pathway consists of a multidisciplinary preoperative evaluation that includes sleep and general medical screening, diagnostic sleep apnea testing, and anatomy phenotyping with physical examination and sedated endoscopy (**Fig. 2**). After completion of the informed consent process, appropriate candidates undergo outpatient surgical implantation of the hardware system as described in the next section. The device is activated in the office setting 4 weeks post implant. The patient then begins nightly therapy use during an initial accommodation period that includes gradual self-titration through a preset range of parameters to optimize comfort as well as symptom improvement. As with any OSA medical device therapy, close clinical follow-up is recommended to assess therapy adherence and patient-reported outcome measures, including an objective adherence report downloaded from the device.

At this juncture, the patient completes postoperative sleep testing either with home portable monitoring or in-laboratory polysomnography to assess objective outcome measures. Once adequate adherence and results have been achieved, the patient is transitioned to a longitudinal management plan across the life of the device (expected battery life >10 years). For patients struggling with inadequate therapy adherence or persistent symptoms or AHI elevation, troubleshooting guidelines are being

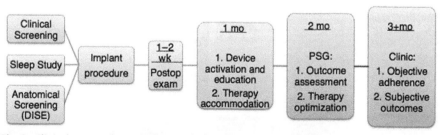

Fig. 2. Clinical care pathway before and after HNS system implantation. After clinical, polysomnographic, and anatomic screening, qualified candidates undergo device implantation, most commonly as an outpatient. At 1 month postoperative, the device is activated and patient starts using the therapy. After another month of therapy accommodation and self-titration at home, patients undergo postoperative sleep testing (1) to assess objective outcome measures and (2) to further titrate therapy and optimize settings for transition to long-term management. PSG, polysomnography.

developed to provide a systematic best-practice approach to optimizing outcomes. Furthermore, as with any OSA treatment plan, multimodality therapy can be used (weight loss, positional therapy, surgical modifications, oral appliance therapy, or other adjunctive treatments) to further augment HNS therapy effectiveness.

SURGICAL IMPLANTATION
Intraoperative Technique

The current FDA-approved device (Inspire Medical Systems, Minneapolis, MN) implantation consists of a 2-hour to 3-hour outpatient procedure performed under general anesthesia.[29] (**Fig. 3**). Fine-wire electrodes are placed in the genioglossus muscle and the hyoglossus/styloglossus muscle complex for intraoperative nerve monitoring. After standard sterile skin preparation and draping, a small incision is made preferably in the right upper neck, parallel to a natural skin crease between the mandible and hyoid. With the submandibular gland retracted posteriorly, tendon of digastric muscle retracted inferiorly, and the mylohyoid muscle retracted anteriorly, the hypoglossal nerve can be identified in its usual location in the floor of the submandibular triangle. Anatomic landmarks, intraoperative nerve monitoring, and direct visualization of tongue motion are all used to selectively identify the distal nerve branches responsible for anterior tongue displacement: branches to the oblique fibers of the genioglossus, the horizontal branches of the genioglossus, and the geniohyoid. All tongue retractor branches are excluded from the cuff electrode so that stimulation produces brisk, forward, uninhibited protrusion of a stiffened tongue (**Fig. 4**).

A second incision is made in the ipsilateral upper chest with creation of a subcutaneous pocket overlying the pectoralis fascia for placement of the implantable pulse generator (IPG). A third incision is made in the ipsilateral lateral chest for placement of the pleural respiratory sensor. The respiratory sensor is inserted between the external and internal intercostal muscles of the underlying intercostal space, with the sensor facing the pleura. The respiratory sensing lead and the stimulation lead are each anchored and then subcutaneously tunneled into the chest pocket for connection to the IPG.

A sterile telemetry unit is then brought into the surgical field and connected to the IPG. Electrical testing is performed to ensure normal impedance values, favorable tongue motion, and an adequate respiratory waveform signal. Confirmation of a good sensing waveform as well as visual and electrical confirmation of uninhibited

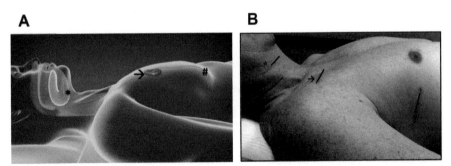

Fig. 3. Implantable HNS system overview. The current FDA-approved implantable HNS system consists of 3 implanted components (A) associated with 3 skin incisions (B), respectively: a stimulation cuff electrode on the distal protrusor branches of the hypoglossal nerve in the right submandibular space (*asterisk*), a subcutaneous pulse generator in the ipsilateral upper chest just inferior to the clavicle (→), and a respiratory sensor in an intercostal space of the ipsilateral lateral chest wall (#). (Images courtesy of Inspire Medical Systems.)

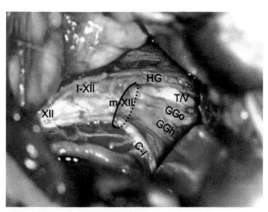

Fig. 4. Distal branching pattern of the hypoglossal nerve (XII). The circle indicates the position of the electrode placement, including m-XII branches (T/V, GGo, GGh), and C-1 in the electrode while excluding I-XII retractor branches (HG). C-1, first cervical nerve; GGh and GGo, fibers to genioglossus muscle horizontal and oblique; HG, fibers to hyoglossus muscle; I-XII, lateral branches of the hypoglossal nerve; m-XII, medial branches of the hypoglossal nerve; T/V, fibers to transverse and vertical intrinsic muscles. (*From* Heiser C, Thaler E, Soose RJ, et al. Technical tips during implantation of selective upper airway stimulation. Laryngoscope 2018;128(3):756-62; with permission.)

tongue protrusion and stiffness is critical to surgical success. All incisions are then copiously irrigated and closed in a multilayer fashion with pressure dressings applied.

Postoperative Management

Postoperatively, radiographs of the neck and chest are obtained to document baseline device position and to rule out electrode displacement or pneumothorax. Because the implant procedure is subcutaneous and does not involve airway surgery, postoperative airway edema and risk are significantly reduced compared with traditional sleep apnea surgeries. In addition, because preoperative screening eliminates significantly obese patients and postoperative opioid requirement is rare, the procedure can be safely performed as an outpatient (same day surgery) in most cases.

Adverse Events

Potential surgical adverse events include bleeding, infection (including the need for device explantation), hematoma/seroma, injury or weakness of the hypoglossal or marginal mandibular nerves, and pneumothorax. Potential therapy-related side effects also are discussed with the patient preoperatively, including tongue abrasion or discomfort, sleep disturbance or insomnia due to stimulation, and inadequate therapy response. Tongue abrasion or soreness are the most common therapy-related nonserious side effects; however, serious adverse events, procedure or therapy related, have been very uncommon in published literature.[21,25] Furthermore, the device implantation procedure and the use of the therapy do not appear to adversely affect swallowing function.[30]

Current Technology Limitations

Unlike nonsurgical medical device treatments, such as positive pressure therapy, HNS implantation requires the use of a general anesthetic as well as 3 external incisions. Although strict MRI incompatibility was an issue with the first FDA-approved Inspire device, the current generation implantable system offers conditional MRI use for head and extremity imaging. Current generator battery life is estimated at 10 to 12 years, which means patients will need to consider future revision surgery or battery replacement or alternative treatments when the battery expires. Technology development is ongoing with efforts to produce a smaller MRI-compatible generator, reduce operative time, improve battery life, incorporate the respiratory sensor into the generator, optimize comfort features, and develop more sophisticated and comprehensive data-monitoring software.

FUTURE CLINICAL DIRECTIONS
Predictors of Therapy Success

With the HNS therapy population now in the thousands and growing rapidly, understanding predictors of therapy response and improving patient selection are critical to long-term success. Using traditional AHI definitions of treatment success, large studies suggest increasing age, decreasing BMI, and female gender are associated with increased likelihood of HNS therapy success.[31,32] Despite the published inverse correlation between outcomes and BMI, a multicenter retrospective review found no difference in postoperative AHI, oxygen desaturation nadir, subjective daytime sleepiness, or success rates in patients with BMI greater than 32 kg/m^2 when compared with those with BMI less than 32 kg/m^2, suggesting that select patients with an elevated BMI can still be successfully treated with HNS therapy.[33] Advances in anatomic and physiologic endotyping using clinical, radiographic, endoscopic, and/ or polysomnographic markers have the potential to strengthen patient selection criteria and bolster outcomes.

Therapy Troubleshooting and Optimization

Postimplant therapy management will play an increasingly important role in the successful longitudinal care of HNS patients, particularly as this treatment modality becomes more accepted and widespread globally. Although many HNS patients are straightforward therapy responders (or even clear nonresponders), there is a substantial population subset with suboptimal clinical response and outcomes, similar to that reported with CPAP or other medical device treatments. Some patients achieve adequate AHI reduction and symptomatic response, but struggle with inadequate adherence or comfort with therapy. Other patients demonstrate excellent therapy adherence, but fail to achieve adequate disease control with residual AHI elevation and/or OSA-related symptoms.

Advanced electrical programming (eg, amplitude, pulse width, rate, electrode configuration) can be systematically analyzed and modified in the outpatient setting, with or without concurrent upper airway endoscopy, to improve long-term outcomes. As clinically indicated, the addition of positional therapy, weight management, lowering of nasal resistance, mandibular repositioning, upper airway surgery, and other adjunctive measures may provide an opportunity to further strengthen HNS outcomes. In summary, for HNS patients with partial but incomplete response, development of standardized best-practice approaches to therapy troubleshooting and modifications are under way and could make a significant difference in long-term outcomes moving forward.

Bigger Data: Adherence and Outcome of Upper Airway Stimulation for Obstructive Sleep Apnea International Registry

The ADHERE registry (Adherence and Outcome of Upper Airway Stimulation for OSA International Registry) was established in 2016 to collect data on HNS therapy patients across multiple US and European sites (**Fig. 5**). Published outcomes from the first 300 registry patients demonstrated mean ± standard deviation AHI decreasing from 35.6 ± 15.3 preoperatively to 10.2 ± 12.9 events per hour postoperatively (P < .001) with accompanying decrease in ESS and mean therapy utilization of 6.5 hours per night.[34] At the time of article submission, more than 1600 patients at more than 40 sites across the United States and Germany are included in the registry thus far, representing the largest cohort of patients studied with HNS therapy to date.[35]

Relationship with Pharyngeal Surgery

Early in the STAR Trial, the question was raised whether prior uvulopalatopharyngo-plasty (UPPP) would improve outcomes with HNS therapy and perhaps even be a prerequisite to successful HNS outcomes. This hypothesis was nullified as the 17% of STAR Trial participants with prior UPPP had similar outcomes to the 83% of participants without prior UPPP.[21] The ADHERE registry also examined whether prior pharyngeal surgery (eg, palatoplasty, excisional tongue base surgery, hyoid suspension) was associated with HNS treatment efficacy, with the investigators similarly reporting no differences in outcome measures in patients with or without prior pharyngeal sleep apnea surgery.[36]

A retrospective analysis of patients undergoing transoral robotic tongue base surgery (TORS) versus HNS implantation at one institution reported significant differences in outcomes between the two, with OSA-related outcome measures, length of hospital stay, and readmission rates all favoring HNS therapy. The investigators reported "surgical success" rates of 86% for HNS versus 54% for TORS, and "cure" rates of 59% for HNS versus 21% for TORS.[37] Similarly, a single-center retrospective review comparing outcomes of expansion sphincter pharyngoplasty (modified UPPP) with HNS therapy reported overall comparable outcomes between the two, trending toward improved AHI reduction and higher success rates with HNS.[38] These studies suggest that HNS therapy may be appropriately used as an effective alternative to pharyngeal surgery rather than just a salvage option after failed pharyngeal surgery. A need exists to develop treatment algorithms and clinical care pathways to assist clinicians in treatment decision-making when faced with CPAP-intolerant patients in need of an effective alternative.

Pediatric Down Syndrome

Although OSA is thought to affect 1% to 5% of the general pediatric population, the prevalence of OSA in children with Down syndrome (DS) is approximately 55% to 90% with severe OSA (AHI >10) affecting almost half of the DS population.[39] A number of pathophysiologic factors, including midface hypoplasia, mandibular deficiency,

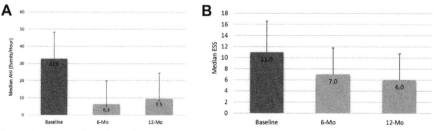

Fig. 5. Outcomes data from the ADHERE Registry. Median AHI (*A*) and ESS (*B*) measurements at baseline and at 6 and 12 months postoperatively. Using Sher criteria on patients with baseline and follow-up AHI data, 83% (n = 485/582) and 69% (n = 265/381) of participants met treatment success after 6 and 12 months, respectively.

relative macroglossia, and hypotonia, all contribute to the increased prevalence. With high rates of congenital heart disease and early-onset dementia, children with DS may be even more vulnerable to the neurocognitive and cardiovascular effects of untreated OSA. Furthermore, CPAP adherence rates remain poor in this population, and approximately 40% of children with DS still have moderate to severe OSA after adenotonsillectomy.[40]

In 2015, the first pediatric HNS implant was performed in a 14-year-old with DS, asthma, congenital heart disease, chronic tracheostomy dependence, and severe refractory OSA despite prior adenotonsillectomy, lingual tonsillectomy, and CPAP trials. HNS therapy resulted in an AHI reduction from 48.5 preoperatively (with capped tracheostomy) to 3.4 postoperatively, leading to successful tracheostomy decannulation and long-term OSA management.[41] An additional 5 adolescent patients with DS were subsequently treated with similar successful OSA outcomes, good patient accommodation and adherence, and low rate of adverse events, results that served as the genesis of the first multicenter pediatric DS trial of HNS therapy.[42] Reports of the first 20 participants in the pediatric DS trial demonstrated 2-month polysomnography data with a median AHI reduction of 85% (interquartile range 75%–92%).[43] The multicenter DS trial is ongoing at the time of this article but early results are very promising that HNS may provide a safe and effective alternative for a pediatric DS population often in desperate need of effective OSA treatment. More studies are needed to assess long-term outcomes as these children grow and transition to adulthood, as well as to determine whether other neuromuscular, congenital, or syndromic subpopulations of patients with OSA could similarly benefit from HNS therapy.

Alternative Device Treatments

Although the Inspire II device is the only implantable upper airway neurostimulation device that is, FDA approved at present, several additional devices show promise in ongoing clinical trials. ImThera Medical (ImThera Medical Inc., San Diego, CA) places multiple stimulating electrodes around the proximal hypoglossal nerve, targeting specific fibers of the nerve.[44] This system interposes rest intervals by sequentially stimulating sectors of the hypoglossal nerve trunk with discrete contacts. The cuff electrode remains continuously activated, thereby eliminating the need for placement of a respiratory sensor. In a 14-patient series, Mwenge and colleagues[19] demonstrated a significant improvement in mean AHI at 12 months, with 2 participants with transient tongue paresis but no additional adverse events. Another system, Nyxoah (Gilde Healthcare, Mon-Saint-Guibert, Belgium) is instead implanted submentally to stimulate distal branches of hypoglossal nerve bilaterally.[45] The implanted stimulator is controlled by an activation chip and external power source placed under the chin via disposable adhesive patch nightly. The system is then activated during sleep and the power source removed from the chin during wakefulness. Early results show improvement in OSA metrics and prospective trials are under way.

DISCLOSURE

Dr R.J. Soose reports research/grant support: Inspire Medical Systems; consultant: Smith & Nephew, Cryosa Inc, Invicta Medical, Galvani Bioelectronics, Enhale Medical, and Inspire Medical Systems. Dr R. Whelan has no conflicts of interest to disclose.

REFERENCES

1. Kushida CA, Nichols DA, Holmes TH, et al. Effects of continuous positive airway pressure on neurocognitive function in obstructive sleep apnea patients: The

Apnea Positive Pressure Long-term Efficacy Study (APPLES). Sleep 2012;35(12): 1593–602.

2. Rosen CL, Auckley D, Benca R, et al. A multisite randomized trial of portable sleep studies and positive airway pressure autotitration versus laboratory-based polysomnography for the diagnosis and treatment of obstructive sleep apnea: The HomePAP Study. Sleep 2012;35(6):757–67.

3. McEvoy RD, Antic NA, Heeley E, et al. CPAP for prevention of cardiovascular events in OSA. N Engl J Med 2016;375:919–31.

4. Pliska BT, Chen H, Lowe AA, et al. OSA and mandibular advancement splints: occlusal effects and progression of changes associated with a decade of treatment. J Clin Sleep Med 2014;10:1285–91.

5. Weaver EM, Maynard C, Yueh B. Survival of veterans with sleep apnea: continuous positive airway pressure versus surgery. Otolaryngol Head Neck Surg 2004;130(6):659–65.

6. Li H-Y. Palatal surgery for obstructive sleep apnea. Sleep Med Clin 2019; 14(1):51–8.

7. Pirklbauer K, Russmueller G, Stiebellehner L, et al. Maxillomandibular advancement for treatment of obstructive sleep apnea syndrome: a systematic review. J Oral Maxillofac Surg 2011;69(6):e165–76.

8. Dempsey JA, Xie A, Patz DS, et al. Physiology in medicine: OSA pathogenesis and treatment – considerations beyond airway anatomy. J Appl Physiol 2014; 116:3–12.

9. White DP. Pathogenesis of obstructive and central sleep apnea. Am J Respir Crit Care Med 2005;172:1363–70.

10. Ragab SM, El Din B, Hefny MA, et al. Hypoglossal nerve conduction studies in patients with obstructive sleep apnea. Egypt J Otolaryngol 2013;29:176–81.

11. Oliven A, Tov N, Geitini L, et al. Effect of genioglossus contraction on pharyngeal lumen and airflow in sleep apnoea patients. Eur Resp J 2007;30:748–58.

12. Oliven A, Odeh M, Geitini L, et al. Effect of coactivation of tongue protrusor and retractor muscles on pharyngeal lumen and airflow in sleep apnea patients. J Appl Physiol 2007;103(5):1662–8.

13. Mu L, Sanders I. Human tongue neuroanatomy: nerve supply and motor endplates. Clin Anat 2010;23:777–91.

14. Sanders I, Mu L. A three-dimensional atlas of human tongue muscles. Anat Rec 2013;296:1102–14.

15. Bassiri Gharb B, Tadisina KK, Rampazzo A, et al. Microsurgical anatomy of the terminal hypoglossal nerve relevant for neurostimulation in obstructive sleep apnea. Neuromodulation 2015. https://doi.org/10.1111/ner.12347.

16. Safiruddin F, Vanderveken OM, de Vries N, et al. Effect of upper-airway stimulation for obstructive sleep apnoea on airway dimensions. Eur Respir J 2015;45(1): 129–38.

17. Eastwood PR, Barnes M, Walsh JH, et al. Treating obstructive sleep apnea with hypoglossal nerve stimulation. Sleep 2011;34:1479–86.

18. Kezirian EJ, Goding GS, Malhotra A, et al. Hypoglossal nerve stimulation improves obstructive sleep apnea: 12-month outcomes. J Sleep Res 2014;23: 77–83.

19. Mwenge GB, Rombaux P, Dury M, et al. Targeted hypoglossal neurostimulation for obstructive sleep apnoea: a 1-year pilot study. Eur Resp J 2013;41:360–7.

20. Van de Heyning PH, Badr MS, Baskin JZ, et al. Implanted upper airway stimulation device for obstructive sleep apnea. Laryngoscope 2012;122:1626–33.

21. Strollo PJ, Soose RJ, Maurer JT, et al. Upper-airway stimulation for obstructive sleep apnea. N Engl J Med 2014;370(2):139–49.
22. Soose RJ, Woodson BT, Gillespie MB, et al. Upper airway stimulation for obstructive sleep apnea: self-reported outcomes at 24 months. J Clin Sleep Med 2016; 12:43–8.
23. Woodson BT, Soose RJ, Gillespie MB, et al. Three-year outcomes of cranial nerve stimulation for obstructive sleep apnea. Otolaryngol Head Neck Surg 2016; 154(1):181–8.
24. Woodson BT, Strohl KP, Soose RJ, et al. Upper airway stimulation for obstructive sleep apnea: 5-year outcomes. Otolaryngol Head Neck Surg 2018;159(1): 194–202.
25. Kent DT, Lee JJ, Strollo PJ Jr, et al. Upper airway stimulation for OSA: early adherence and outcome results of one center. Otolaryngol Head Neck Surg 2016. https://doi.org/10.1177/0194599816636619.
26. Certal VF, Zaghi S, Riaz M, et al. Hypoglossal nerve stimulation in the treatment of obstructive sleep apnea: a systematic review and meta-analysis. Laryngoscope 2015;125(5):1254–64.
27. Huntley C, Kaffenberger T, Doghramji K, et al. Upper airway stimulation for treatment of obstructive sleep apnea: an evaluation and comparison of outcomes at two academic centers. J Clin Sleep Med 2017;13(9):1075–9.
28. Heiser C, Maurer JT, Hofauer B, et al. Outcomes of upper airway stimulation for obstructive sleep apnea in a multicenter German postmarket study. Otolaryngol Head Neck Surg 2017;156(2):378–84.
29. Heiser C, Thaler E, Boon M, et al. Updates of operative techniques for upper airway stimulation. Laryngoscope 2016;126:S12–6.
30. Huntley C, Vasconcellos A, Mullen M, et al. The impact of upper airway stimulation on swallowing function. Ear Nose Throat J 2019;98(8):496–9.
31. Withrow K, Evans S, Harwick J, et al. Upper airway stimulation response in older adults with moderate to severe obstructive sleep apnea. Otolaryngol Head Neck Surg 2019;161(4):714–9.
32. Heiser C, Steffen A, Boon M, et al. Post-approval upper airway stimulation predictors of treatment effectiveness in the ADHERE registry. Eur Resp J 2019;53(1) [pii: 1801405].
33. Huntley C, Steffen A, Doghramji K, et al. Upper airway stimulation in patients with obstructive sleep apnea and an elevated body mass index: a multi-institutional review. Laryngoscope 2018;128(10):2425–8.
34. Boon M, Huntley C, Steffen A, et al. Upper airway stimulation for obstructive sleep apnea: results from the ADHERE registry. Otolaryngol Head Neck Surg 2018; 159(2):379–85.
35. Thaler E, Schwab R, Maurer J, et al. Results of the ADHERE upper airway stimulation registry and predictors of therapy efficacy. Laryngoscope 2019. https://doi.org/10.1002/lary.28286.
36. Kezirian EJ, Heiser C, Steffen A, et al. Previous surgery and hypoglossal nerve stimulation for obstructive sleep apnea. Otolaryngol Head Neck Surg 2019; 161(5):897–903.
37. Huntley C, Topf MC, Christopher V, et al. Comparing upper airway stimulation to transoral robotic base of tongue resection for treatment of obstructive sleep apnea. Laryngoscope 2019;129(4):1010–3.
38. Huntley C, Chou DW, Doghramji K, et al. Comparing upper airway stimulation to expansion sphincter pharyngoplasty: a single university experience. Ann Otol Rhinol Laryngol 2018;127(6):379–83.

39. Chamseddin BH, Johnson RF, Mitchell RB. OSA in children with Down syndrome: demographic, clinical, and polysomnographic features. Otolaryngol Head Neck Surg 2019;160:150–7.
40. Farhood Z, Isley JW, Ong AA. Adenotonsillectomy outcomes in patients with Down syndrome and OSA. Laryngoscope 2017;127:1465–70.
41. Diercks GR, Keamy D, Kinane TB, et al. Hypoglossal nerve stimulator implantation in an adolescent with Down syndrome and sleep apnea. Pediatrics 2016; 137(5) [pii:e2015366].
42. Diercks GR, Wentland C, Keamy D, et al. Hypoglossal nerve stimulation in adolescents with Down syndrome and OSA. JAMA Otolaryngol Head Neck Surg 2017. [Epub ahead of print].
43. Caloway CL, Diercks GR, Keamy D, et al. Update on hypoglossal nerve stimulation in children with Down syndrome and obstructive sleep apnea. Laryngoscope 2018;144:37–42. https://doi.org/10.1002/lary.28138.
44. Fleury Curado T, Oliven A, Sennes LU, et al. Neurostimulation treatment of OSA. Chest 2018;154(6):1435–47.
45. Eastwood PR, Barnes M, MacKay SG, et al. Bilateral hypoglossal nerve stimulation for treatment of adult obstructive sleep apnoea. Eur Resp J 2020;55(1) [pii: 1901320].

Skeletal Surgery for Obstructive Sleep Apnea

Michael Awad, MD, FRCSC[a], Robson Capasso, MD[b],*

KEYWORDS

- Maxillomandibular advancement • Genioglossus advancement • DOME
- Distraction osteogenesis • Maxillary expansion • Dentofacial deformity
- Retrognathia • Micrognathia

KEY POINTS

- Skeletal surgery originated with the procedures of maxillomandibular advancement (MMA) and genioglossus advancement (GGA). These techniques originated from a need for an effective multilevel surgical technique that did not have the associated comorbidity of tracheostomy in patients with severe OSA.
- Operative technique and perioperative care related to MMA surgery have consistently improved, leading to improved reliability and patient outcomes.
- The central role of skeletal surgery in the revised Stanford protocol is a theme of the article, with the role of these procedures as functioning in a continuum with other surgical techniques, such as palatopharyngoplasty, upper airway stimulation, and of course medical management.
- This article focuses on the role of skeletal surgery within the modified Stanford protocol with particular attention focused on the evolved role of MMA. First, surgery in patients presenting with congenital dentofacial deformity or characteristic drug-induced sleep endoscopy findings, then the growing role of maxillary expansion in a newly identified patient phenotype, and finally genioglossus advancement, are discussed.

BACKGROUND

Skeletal surgery has played a central role in the surgical management of obstructive sleep apnea (OSA) since the first reported case of isolated mandibular advancement for OSA at our center in 1984.[1] Skeletal surgery originated with the procedures of maxillomandibular advancement (MMA) and genioglossus advancement (GGA). These techniques originated from a need for an effective multilevel surgical technique that did not have the associated comorbidity of tracheostomy in patients with severe OSA.

[a] Division of Sleep Surgery, Department of Otolaryngology–Head & Neck Surgery, Northwestern University, 675 N, St Clair Street, 15th Floor, Suite 200, Chicago, IL 60611, USA;
[b] Division of Sleep Surgery, Department of Otolaryngology–Head & Neck Surgery, Stanford University, 801 Welch Road, Stanford, CA 94305, USA
* Corresponding author.
E-mail address: rcapasso@stanford.edu

Otolaryngol Clin N Am 53 (2020) 459–468
https://doi.org/10.1016/j.otc.2020.02.008
0030-6665/20/© 2020 Elsevier Inc. All rights reserved.

oto.theclinics.com

Since then, the role of skeletal surgery has involved to include bi-jaw advancement techniques, maxillary expansion, and genioglossus advancement among others. The number of publications on these procedures has been increasing over the past 10 years as per a recent meta-analysis by Awad and colleagues[2] Operative technique and perioperative care related to MMA surgery has consistently improved, leading to improved reliability and patient outcomes.[3–5]

The central role of skeletal surgery in the revised Stanford protocol is a theme of the article, with the role of these procedures as functioning in a continuum with other surgical techniques, such as palatopharyngoplasty, upper airway stimulation, and of course medical management (**Fig. 1**).

This article focuses on the role of skeletal surgery within the modified Stanford protocol with particular attention focused on the evolved role of MMA. First, surgery in patients presenting with congenital dentofacial deformity or characteristic drug-induced sleep endoscopy findings, then the growing role of maxillary expansion in a newly

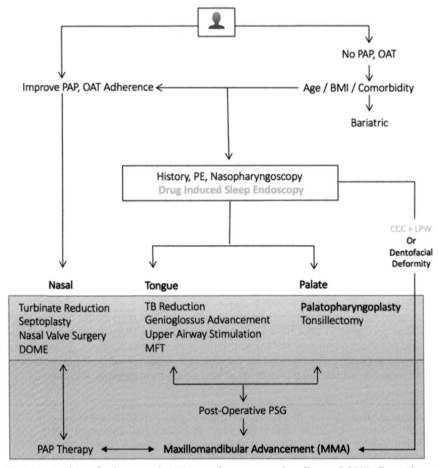

Fig. 1. Revised Stanford protocol. CCC, complete concentric collapse; DOME, distraction osteogenesis maxillary expansion; LPW, lateral pharyngeal wall; MFT, myofunctional therapy; OAT, oral appliance therapy; PAP, positive airway pressure; PE, physical examination; PSG, polysomongraph. (*From* Liu SY-C, Awad M, Riley R, et al. The role of the revised Stanford protocol in today's precision medicine. Sleep Med Clin. 2019;14(1):103; with permission.)

identified patient phenotype, and finally genioglossus advancement, are discussed. Less commonly used and validated techniques, such as isolated mandibular advancement and maxillomandibular expansion are not discussed in this article.

CLINICAL EXAMINATION

Patient selection has improved with the widespread acceptance of a drug-induced sleep endoscopy as a diagnostic tool in the preoperative evaluation of surgical patients with OSA. However, selection for skeletal surgery remains rooted in clinical examination and phenotypical patient characteristics.

Traditionally, selection for skeletal surgery involves a comprehensive medical history and physical examination, head and neck examination (with fiberoptic laryngoscopy), cephalometry, and polysomnography. With the advent of virtual surgical planning (VSP), most patients forego lateral cephalometry in favor of noncontrast fine-cut maxillofacial computed tomography scanning with 3-dimensional reconstructions. This allows for a direct and easily accessible visual assessment of anteroposterior airway space as well as assessment of congenital dentofacial deformity.

In patients undergoing drug-induced sleep endoscopy, severe lateral pharyngeal wall collapse with circumferential concentric collapse at the level of the velum was identified as a predictor of surgical success in patients who undergo MMA as a primary procedure.[6–8]

With the advent of VSP, GGA has evolved from the traditionally described rectangular osteotomy of the lower mandible into a patient-specific procedure THAT takes into account individual anatomy to optimize functional and cosmetic outcomes. The role of VSP in modern skeletal surgery for OSA is discussed in detail in the "Maxillomandibular advancement" and "Genioglossus advancement" sections below.

GENIOGLOSSUS ADVANCEMENT/GENIOPLASTY

Longstanding electromyographic studies have demonstrated the role of the genioglossus muscle as the major pharyngeal dilator musculature of the airway during sleep. Its role has been extensively implicated in the pathophysiology of OSA with the rationale that upper airway collapse occurs as a result of failure of the dilator muscles of the airway to sustain patency during the respiratory cycle.[9,10]

Traditionally, GGA has played a role in multilevel airway management of the patient with OSA. The term multilevel refers to treatment involving more than 1 airway site in 1 individual patient. This typically refers to the nasal airway, nasopharynx, retropalatal space, tongue base, and/or hypopharynx. In combination with nasal and palate procedures (the originally described Stanford "phase 1"), this multilevel surgical approach has demonstrated a 66% surgical success rate, with GGA conferring a 10% improvement in surgical success.[11] However, appropriate patient selection as it relates to predictability of outcome remains an area of uncertainty in preoperative evaluation for GGA. Genioglossus tension as measured by tensiometry has been used to predict postoperative response. Decreased tension and increased mandibular width were demonstrated as positive predictive factors for surgical success.

Infrequently, isolated GGA is used in patients demonstrating exclusively tongue base collapse. Comprehensive meta-analysis by Song and colleagues[12] demonstrated a 43.8% reduction in the apnea-hypopnea index (AHI) for patients who underwent isolated GGA and 43.8% for patients who underwent standard genioplasty.

Confusingly, some authors use the terms "genioglossus advancement" and "genioplasty" interchangeably. For clarity, GGA refers to the technique of advancing the genial tubercle and associated muscles via an osteotomy within the anterior aspect of the mandible. This differs from genioplasty where the genial tubercle is advanced via a horizontal sliding osteotomy.

The core rationale behind performing GGA persists from its original description in 1984. That is, stabilization of the hypopharyngeal airway with anterior movement of the genioglossus complex adding tension to the base of tongue and thereby expanding airway space during sleep.[1]

The procedure was adapted by Riley and Powell to include a superior extension thus capturing the entire genial tubercle. They subsequently revised the procedure to involve a bicortical rectangular osteotomy while maintaining continuity of the inferior mandible border to reduce the risk of mandibular fracture.[13,14]

Patient-specific GGA has led to improved reliability and ease of the procedure.[15] With the use of VSP software making use of a preoperative, noncontrast, maxillofacial computed tomography, the location of the genioglossus complex on the posterior aspect of the mandible is identified along with the canine roots and mental nerve protrusion bilaterally. The planned osteotomy is digitally visualized with care taken to avoid the mental nerves and leave at least 7 to 8 mm of inferior separation from the planned osteotomy to the canine roots while incorporating the genioglossus complex (**Fig. 2**). 3D printed splints, which have traditionally been tooth-borne making use of the patient's dental models, have been used.

The technique has evolved to make use of surgical cutting guides, which are anchored on the inferior mandible border contour negating the need for time-consuming and costly dental models (**Figs. 3** and **4**).

Complications

Intraoperatively, the most worrisome complication is that of avulsion of the genioglossus muscle from its attachment at the posterior mandibular border. In most circumstances this is not correctable and so care should be taken when advancing the osteotomized mandibular segment to avoid excessive traction on the muscle belly.

More common but less severe complications, including persistent paresthesia of the lower lip, wound infection, and injury to the canine tooth roots, are possible, but

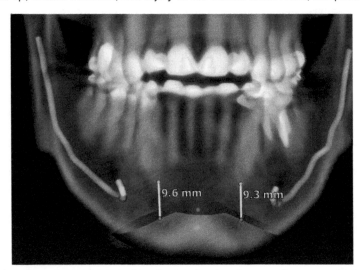

Fig. 2. The planned osteotomy is digitally visualized with care taken to avoid the mental nerves and leave at least 7 to 8 mm of inferior separation from the planned osteotomy to the canine roots while incorporating the genioglossus complex.

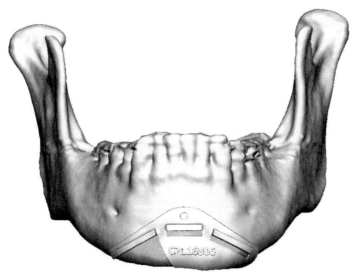

Fig. 3. The technique has evolved to make use of surgical cutting guides which are anchored on the inferior mandible border contour negating the need for time-consuming and costly dental models.

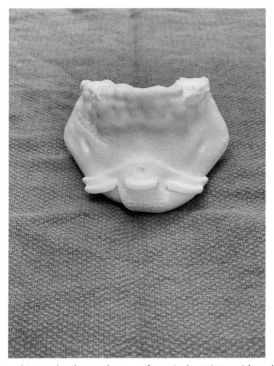

Fig. 4. The technique has evolved to make use of surgical cutting guides which are anchored on the inferior mandible border contour negating the need for time-consuming and costly dental models.

these risks are likely mitigated with the use of the VSP-guided, patient-specific genioplasty described above.

Postoperatively, mandibular fracture can occur, particularly in techniques that violate the inferior mandible border.

SURGICALLY ASSISTED PALATAL EXPANSION

A phenotype of growing interest to the sleep surgeon is the subset of patients with OSA who demonstrate persistent nasal obstruction and a characteristically high-arched, narrow "arch-shaped" hard palate. These patients who have failed nasal surgery (in the form of septoplasty, inferior turbinate reduction, nasal valve repair, and/or endoscopic sinus surgery) have been demonstrated to show consistent skeletal phenotypes. These patients are more likely to demonstrate an acute maxillary angle, narrow maxillary width, and high-arched palate.[16] In other words, patients with persistent nasal obstruction are more likely to demonstrate a narrow, high-arched hard palate.

Rapid maxillary expansion with the use of orthodontic expanders has consistently demonstrated efficacy for treating OSA in the pediatric population,[17] particularly for children who fail adenotonsillectomy.[18,19] With the understanding of how this characteristic maxillary phenotype contributes to nasal obstruction by resulting in increasing nasal airway resistance at the level of the nasal floor, similar principles can be applied to the adult patient with OSA.[20,21]

Patients undergoing palatal expansion can require 12 to 18 months for full orthodontic treatment with closure of the diastema. During bony consolidation of the diastema at the maxillary floor, the maxillary expansion appliance is left in place for 6 to 8 months after expansion.

There are 3 main indications for adult patients with OSA to undergo DOME (distraction osteogenesis maxillary expansion):

1. Patients with OSA presenting with transverse maxillary discrepancy/crossbite
2. Patients with mild OSA or upper airway resistance syndrome demonstrating persistent nasal obstruction in the setting of a narrow, high-arched palate who:
   a. Have previously undergone nasal surgery
   b. Have not previously undergone nasal surgery but do not demonstrate significant septal deviation, inferior turbinate hypertrophy, or nasal valve collapse
3. Patients with moderate to severe OSA as part of a broad treatment plan, including palatopharyngoplasty, upper airway stimulation, or MMA with characteristic maxillary findings of high-arched, narrow palate

Complications

Patients seeking consultation for DOME should be counseled on the risks of asymmetric maxillary expansion, loss of vitality to either central incisor, palatal fistula, and temporary V2 paresthesia.

Minor risks include those of postoperative epistaxis, which is typically self-limiting, and persistent paresthesia at the vestibular incision site.

Palatal expansion does not result in esthetic facial changes despite the increase in area seen at the level of the nasal floor.

MAXILLOMANDIBULAR ADVANCEMENT

Consistently the cornerstone of skeletal surgery for OSA, MMA remains the most effective multilevel procedure available for treatment of OSA, with surgical success and cure rates of 85.5% and 38%, respectively.[5] MMA enlarges the posterior airway space at multiple anatomic sites, including the nasopharynx, oropharynx, and hypopharynx.[22,23]

MMA is a procedure in which both the maxilla and mandible are advanced in an antero-superior direction relative to the airway, thus resulting in increased tension forces on the attached pharyngeal airway muscles to dilate the posterior airway space.

Many evolutionary modifications have accompanied its development to allow optimal movement of the facial skeleton to appropriately treat the airway while delicately balancing facial esthetics.

In previous iterations of the Stanford protocol, phase I surgery as described above was followed by MMA when other multilevel procedures failed to resolve OSA. This "salvage" use of MMA has changed dramatically today, with a proportion of patients opting to undergo upfront MMA as a primary procedure. This has been sparked both by evolutions in technique as well as the use of dynamic assessment in the form of drug-induced sleep endoscopy, which has allowed the identification of airway phenotypes that reliably benefit from an MMA-first approach. That is, those patients who demonstrate lateral pharyngeal wall collapse *and* concentric collapse at the level of the velum are likely to benefit from upfront MMA.[7]

The use of MMA to reduce disease burden (AHI) while attenuating patient symptoms and improving quality of life is a different treatment endpoint from previous descriptions where surgical cure functioned as the primary goal.[11]

When compared with use of optimal continuous positive airway pressure, MMA performs favorably with restoration of normal sleep architecture demonstrated after MMA, particularly in relation to increase in rapid eye movement sleep seen in patients who have undergone the procedure.[24,25]

Anesthetic Considerations

Our extensive experience in airway management of patients with a variety of occlusal inclinations and airway configurations has led to the development of a consistent, reliable protocol for planning of anesthetic considerations in MMA. Patients with OSA undergoing MMA surgery are best suited to undergo intubation with a micro:laryngoscopy tube, as the length of these endotracheal tubes provides sufficient length for the longer airways encountered in patients with OSA. The tube is trimmed leaving 1 cm from the nasal sill and a 120° metal connector used to secure the tube to the anesthetic circuit over the forehead. Care is taken to avoid pressure on the nasal ala, which can lead to necrosis over the duration of the treatment.

Total intravenous anesthesia with agents, such as propofol and remifentanil, are preferred to minimize the use of volatile anesthetic agents. These agents allow for less postoperative nausea, and vomiting, while allowing for rapid emergence.

Controlled hypotension with a mean arterial pressure of 60 mm Hg is preferred to minimize blood loss during surgery, which is typically between 200 and 300 cm³.

Postoperatively, the MMA surgeon should be available to assist anesthesia in a tandem approach to suction the airway nasally during extubation, avoiding the risk of laryngospasm and subsequent need for reintubation or urgent airway intervention.

Operative Technique

Full details of our operative technique are beyond the scope of this article and can be found in our other publications.[26,27]

The advent of VSP has allowed for reliable, predictable planning of facial movements with the creation of an intermediate splint used after surgical creation of LeFort osteotomies. A second, final splint is then used to secure the condylar and dentate segments in their final position after the bilateral sagittal split osteotomy.

It is well established that the degree of maxillary advancement is correlated to surgical success. Counterclockwise rotation (CCW) of the maxilla allows for a greater degree of subsequent mandibular advancement without necessitating unsightly excessive advancement of the maxilla and compromise of nasal form and function. Thus, the *degree* of CCW rotation predicts surgical success.[5,28] CCW rotation can increase the retropalatal length of the uvula while combating inferior positioning of the uvula and decreasing upper airway length.[29] After LeFort I osteotomy and during mobilization of the maxilla, an appropriately sized bony wedge is cut with the use of a reciprocating saw to accommodate the preplanned CCW movement. Care must be taken in planning of maxillary movement to maintain appropriate incisor show and avoiding compromising esthetic balance and smile.

To that end, during maxillary down-fracture nasal form and function is optimized by resecting an inferior portion of the septum as well as reducing the inferior turbinates. Finally, pyriform-plasty with the use of a pineapple burr is performed to expand the nasal aperture and reduce nasal airway resistance while preventing unfavorable cosmetic nasal outcomes.[30]

Complications

With attentive collaboration between the sleep surgeon, the anesthesiologist, and the operating team in addition to meticulous surgical technique and reduced operating times, MMA is safe with a low major complication rate.[31,32]

Malocclusion can occur, which may require revision surgery if orthodontic salvage is unsuccessful.

Nasal obstruction and congestion is expected after surgery, often secondary to nasal sinus drainage, and some degree of epistaxis. This is mitigated with routine nasal saline irrigation upward of 3 times daily in the immediate postoperative period. Seventeen percent of patients undergoing MMA required corrective nasal surgery for functional or cosmetic reasons.[30]

Intraoperatively, during down-fracture of the maxilla, injury to the descending palatine artery(ies) can occur. If the descending palatine artery is injured the proximal segment should be located and ligated. In the rare instance where avascular necrosis of the palate is observed, the maxilla should be resuspended to its original position and the procedure suspended.

Given the significant degree of mandibular advancement (often upward of 15 mm), stretching of the inferior alveolar nerve resulting in V3 paresthesia is common after the sagittal split osteotomy. Most patients have full return of sensation at 6 months. In rare cases the nerve can be severed, and it should be reapproximated with the use of an 8-0 monofilament suture.

Postoperatively, wound dehiscence of the mandibular vestibular incisions is commonly seen and can be treated conservatively with close follow-up, antibiotics, and meticulous oral hygiene when there is no evidence of infection. Approximately 20% to 40% patients have been described to need removal of deep hardware (most commonly mandibular plates) due to persistent low-grade infection. (Take a look at the Blumen, et al,[31] 2016 article for reference).

SUMMARY

Modern nuances combined with novel surgical techniques have dramatically improved the reliability, safety, and precision of skeletal surgical techniques for the treatment of OSA. The use of VSP has allowed for individualized treatment plans that take into account individual patient anatomy mitigating many of the risks associated with traditional GGA. In addition, it has allowed for the evolution of a powerful airway technique that delicately balances facial form and function in the setting of MMA.

DISCLOSURE

The authors have nothing to disclose.

REFERENCES

1. Riley R, Guilleminault C, Powell N, et al. Mandibular osteotomy and hyoid bone advancement for obstructive sleep apnea: a case report. Sleep 1984;7(1):79–82.
2. Awad M, Gouveia C, Zaghi S, et al. Changing practice: trends in skeletal surgery for obstructive sleep apnea. J Craniomaxillofac Surg 2018. https://doi.org/10.1016/j.jcms.2018.11.005.
3. Li KK, Powell NB, Riley RW, et al. Long-term results of maxillomandibular advancement surgery. Sleep Breath 2000;04(03):137–40.
4. Riley RW, Powell NB, Guilleminault C. Maxillofacial surgery and nasal CPAP. A comparison of treatment for obstructive sleep apnea syndrome. Chest 1990; 98(6):1421–5.
5. Zaghi S, Holty J-EC, Certal V, et al. Maxillomandibular advancement for treatment of obstructive sleep apnea. JAMA Otolaryngol Head Neck Surg 2016; 142(1):58–9.
6. Liu SY-C, Huon L-K, Iwasaki T, et al. Efficacy of maxillomandibular advancement examined with drug-induced sleep endoscopy and computational fluid dynamics airflow modeling. Otolaryngol Head Neck Surg 2016;154(1):189–95.
7. Liu SY-C, Huon L-K, Powell NB, et al. Lateral pharyngeal wall tension after maxillomandibular advancement for obstructive sleep apnea is a marker for surgical success: observations from drug-induced sleep endoscopy. J Oral Maxillofac Surg 2015;73(8):1575–82.
8. Awad M, Okland TS, Nekhendzy V. Drug-induced sleep endoscopy. Atlas Oral Maxillofac Surg Clin North Am 2019;27(1):7–10.
9. White DP. Sleep-related breathing disorder. 2. Pathophysiology of obstructive sleep apnoea. Thorax 1995;50(7):797–804.
10. NHLBI Workshop summary. Respiratory muscle fatigue. Report of the Respiratory Muscle Fatigue Workshop Group. Am Rev Respir Dis 1990;142(2):474–80.
11. Liu SY-C, Awad M, Riley R, et al. The role of the revised Stanford protocol in today's precision medicine. Sleep Med Clin 2019;14(1):99–107.
12. Song SA, Chang ET, Certal V, et al. Genial tubercle advancement and genioplasty for obstructive sleep apnea: a systematic review and meta-analysis. Laryngoscope 2017;127(4):984–92.
13. Riley RW, Powell NB, Guilleminault C. Inferior sagittal osteotomy of the mandible with hyoid myotomy-suspension: a new procedure for obstructive sleep apnea. Otolaryngol Head Neck Surg 1986;94(5):589–93.
14. Li KK, Riley RW, Powell NB, et al. Obstructive sleep apnea surgery: genioglossus advancement revisited. J Oral Maxillofac Surg 2001;59(10):1181–4 [discussion: 1185].
15. Liu SY-C, Huon L-K, Zaghi S, et al. An accurate method of designing and performing individual-specific genioglossus advancement. Otolaryngol Head Neck Surg 2017;156(1):194–7.

16. Williams R, Patel V, Chen Y-F, et al. The upper airway nasal complex: structural contribution to persistent nasal obstruction. Otolaryngol Head Neck Surg 2019; 268. 194599819838262.

17. Pirelli P, Saponara M, Guilleminault C. Rapid maxillary expansion (RME) for pediatric obstructive sleep apnea: a 12-year follow-up. Sleep Med 2015;16(8):933–5.

18. Iwasaki T, Takemoto Y, Inada E, et al. The effect of rapid maxillary expansion on pharyngeal airway pressure during inspiration evaluated using computational fluid dynamics. Int J Pediatr Otorhinolaryngol 2014;78(8):1258–64.

19. Iwasaki T, Saitoh I, Takemoto Y, et al. Tongue posture improvement and pharyngeal airway enlargement as secondary effects of rapid maxillary expansion: a cone-beam computed tomography study. Am J Orthod Dentofacial Orthop 2013;143(2):235–45.

20. Vinha PP, Eckeli AL, Faria AC, et al. Effects of surgically assisted rapid maxillary expansion on obstructive sleep apnea and daytime sleepiness. Sleep Breath 2016;20(2):501–8.

21. Abdelwahab M, Yoon A, Okland T, et al. Impact of distraction osteogenesis maxillary expansion on the internal nasal valve in obstructive sleep apnea. Otolaryngol Head Neck Surg 2019;42(3). 194599819842808.

22. Costa E Sousa RA, Santos Gil dos NA. Craniofacial skeletal architecture and obstructive sleep apnoea syndrome severity. J Craniomaxillofac Surg 2013; 41(8):740–6.

23. Camacho M, Liu SY, Certal V, et al. Large maxillomandibular advancements for obstructive sleep apnea: an operative technique evolved over 30 years. J Craniomaxillofac Surg 2015;43(7):1113–8.

24. Liu SYC, Huon LK, Ruoff C, et al. Restoration of sleep architecture after maxillomandibular advancement: success beyond the apnea-hypopnea index. Int J Oral Maxillofac Surg 2017;46(12):1533–8.

25. McArdle N, Devereux G, Heidarnejad H, et al. Long-term use of CPAP therapy for sleep apnea/hypopnea syndrome. Am J Respir Crit Care Med 1999;159(4 Pt 1): 1108–14.

26. Liu SY-C, Awad M, Riley RW. Maxillomandibular advancement: contemporary approach at Stanford. Atlas Oral Maxillofac Surg Clin North Am 2019;27(1): 29–36.

27. Powell NB, Riley RW, Guilleminault C. Maxillofacial surgical techniques for hypopharyngeal obstruction in obstructive sleep apnea. Operat Tech Otolaryngol Head Neck Surg 1991;2(2):112–9.

28. Holty J-EC, Guilleminault C. Maxillomandibular advancement for the treatment of obstructive sleep apnea: a systematic review and meta-analysis. Sleep Med Rev 2010;14(5):287–97.

29. Susarla SM, Abramson ZR, Dodson TB, et al. Upper airway length decreases after maxillomandibular advancement in patients with obstructive sleep apnea. J Oral Maxillofac Surg 2011;69(11):2872–8.

30. Liu SY-C, Lee P-J, Awad M, et al. Corrective nasal surgery after maxillomandibular advancement for obstructive sleep apnea: experience from 379 cases. Otolaryngol Head Neck Surg 2017;157(1):156–9.

31. Blumen MB, Buchet I, Meulien P, et al. Complications/adverse effects of maxillomandibular advancement for the treatment of OSA in regard to outcome. Otolaryngol Head Neck Surg 2009;141(5):591–7.

32. Andrews J, Barrera J. Does tension matter? A comparison of genioglossus advancement using tensiometry to predict successful outcomes. Otolaryngol Head Neck Surg 2011;145(2 Suppl):270.

Printed and bound by CPI Group (UK) Ltd, Croydon, CR0 4YY

03/10/2024

01040400-0012